A FEW OF OUR

Favorite Things

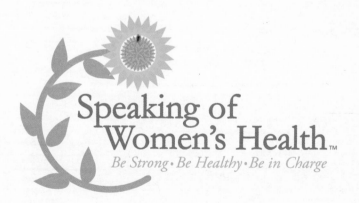

Speaking of Women's Health™

Be Strong · Be Healthy · Be in Charge

THE BOOK   VOLUME VI

Table of Contents

Healthy Recipes

"Me" Time

Family Time

Table of Contents

Healthy Recipes

The nutritional analysis provided is not intended for medical nutritional therapy. If you are following a strict diet for medical or dietary reasons, consult first with a physician or dietitian before planning your meals.

This book is designed to provide information about health, not medical advice. Please consult your physician if you have any questions or concerns.

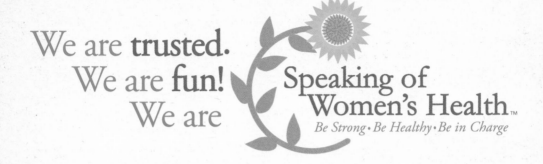

We are **trusted.**
We are **fun!**
We are

Speaking of Women's Health™

Be Strong · Be Healthy · Be in Charge

A Few of Our Favorite Things is the 6th in a series of books we've written for women nationwide and just one of the ways we spread our mission of "educating women to make informed decisions about health, well-being and personal safety for themselves and their families."

Since 1996, Speaking of Women's Health® has been educating and empowering women through more than 50 conferences and events across the country. In addition to our Speaking of Women's Health conferences, we have created Universal Sisters™ for African-American women, Hablando de la Salud de la Mujer® for Hispanic women, Growing Together, Connecting for Life™ for mothers and daughters and, for the men in our lives, Speaking to Men About Health™. We host in-store events at Wal-Mart stores nationwide — and have free health brochures in Wal-Mart stores every day. We also produce a free quarterly newsletter and a free monthly e-newsletter.

Through our Web site, **www.speakingofwomenshealth.com**, you can find health information on topics from healthy eating to exercise, and from beauty to self-esteem — just to name a few! You'll also find videos on a variety of women's health topics, as well as healthy and delicious recipes.

A Note from Our Founder...

As you look through this book,
you will no doubt identify with some of the "favorite things" these female leaders and celebrities have shared. While some favorites are treasured heirlooms, children's "creations," bits of glamour, books or music... the things we most like to see, hold or listen to; there are other intangible favorites that we embrace with our hearts and minds. On the following pages, I have shared a few of the things that make my heart sing. As women, we not only respond to our five senses, we also respond to our sixth sense — that voice inside us that tells us "go ahead, take a chance... this is the right thing to do!" Speaking of Women's Health became my intangible favorite... my "ah–ha moment," inspired by the idea of sharing with other women. At that moment, I knew that my mission in life was to bring together women across America, talented experts and brilliant physicians. Imagine how thrilled I was that our sponsoring companies and brands saw this as a wonderful way to respond to women's needs and support our mission "to educate women to make informed decisions about health, well-being and personal safety for themselves and their families."

One of my favorite things has been connecting with all of you. You have guided Speaking of Women's Health to give you what you want to hear, when and where you want to hear it. It has been written that Speaking of Women's Health uniquely understands the psychology of women. We do, because you have told us what information is most important to you.

I sincerely hope that Speaking of Women's Health is one of your favorite things. As our Web site is taking on a greater importance, women nationwide are bookmarking our site as a favorite. I hope we are your trusted resource for current health information and a place to turn to find humor, joy and compassion and a place to share your wisdom. And now, we feature "Healthy Conversations," our new blog, letting you connect with women throughout the country. Plus, we give you the opportunity to make your voice heard through "Speak Out." Log on to **www.speakingofwomenshealth.com**.

As always, Speaking of Women's Health is here for you. Whether it's finding a healthy weight, having strong bones, being heart healthy, preparing for a new baby, strengthening your personal relationships or enhancing your self-esteem through your inner and outer beauty... Speaking of Women's Health is ALL ABOUT YOU!

Warm wishes to you and your loved ones,

Dianne

Dianne Dunkelman, *Founder & CEO, Speaking of Women's Health*

A FEW OF MY
Favorite Things

Sophia and Henry, the sweetest
children in the world

My favorite chair in a favorite
corner of my house

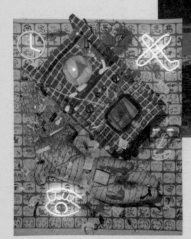

"I See Time Fly" by Nam Jun Paik,
the father of video art

Here's my fashion
icon, everybody has
one, you know

One of my greatest honors...
the seal and the key to the city of
Cincinnati, my home town

Learning to "txt"...
good 4 U & me 2.
XOXO
sweet dreams

veri_on

‣ 1X INBOX – OPEN ◄

What do i say?, but i
am blessed w you

Jan 5. 10:03 pm

rase   REPLY Options

Words to live by, I give this book to people I love

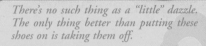

There's no such thing as a "little" dazzle. The only thing better than putting these shoes on is taking them off.

Dianne Dunkelman

Founder and Chief Executive Officer ~ Speaking of Women's Health

Getting back in the swing of my favorite sport. Tennis anyone?

"Paris" by Yves St. Laurent. The only fragrance I ever wear.

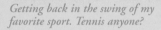

My kids always call me "Super Mom" when I carry a red purse

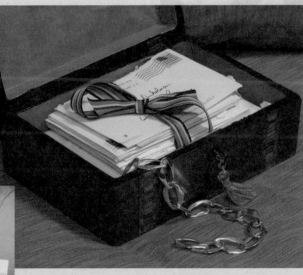

Love notes nestled in an antique box. The saved letters, the beautiful box and the necklace all arrived as a gift. Gives a new meaning to "chain letters."

7

A FEW OF

Your Favorite Things

After you've had a chance to read this book and enjoy some of the "favorites" that other women have shared, we hope you will consider using this space to think about and list some of your "favorite" things.

We were so touched by Lisa Peterson's letter (see page 121) describing what this project meant to her, we decided to dedicate a place for you to experience your own favorites. Maybe you'll even be inspired to take some pictures, put them in an envelope and tuck them into this book.

_____

_____

_____

_____

_____

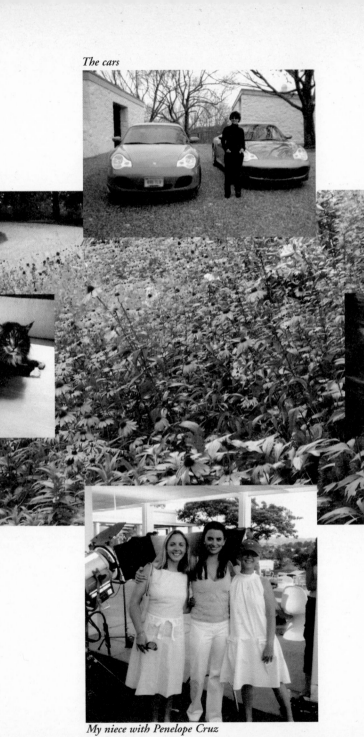

The cars

*Venus,
the cat*

*Ruby,
the cat*

My niece with Penelope Cruz

A FEW OF MY
Favorite Things

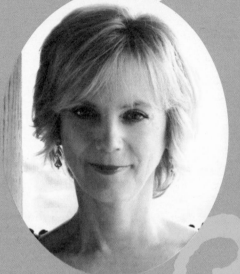

Carol Hamilton

President ~ L'Oreal Paris

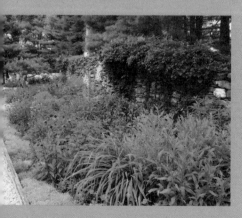

Carol sent us 13 pictures of her glorious gardens in the country. It's clear that as the president of L'Oreal Paris, she's all about beauty. No surprise to us. As Carol says, "Inner beauty is equally important as outer beauty."

Put Your Best Face Forward

If one of your mother's favorite sayings is,
"Beauty is more than skin deep," by now you know she is right!
Pretty is as pretty does... so start "doing" today.

Be kind and considerate, think positive thoughts, maintain your spirituality, know that you are unique, special and precious and you will have inner beauty. You can begin your outer beauty today, by taking some of this advice for beautiful skin.

Daily Skincare Prescription

You can have healthy-looking skin by investing just 4 minutes, 2 times every day, on your skincare routine. Combining proper skincare, eating right, exercising and managing stress gives you a more complete regimen.

Extra Tip

The skin on your neck and chest is delicate and develops the unwanted signs of aging just like your face. Be sure to cleanse, tone, moisturize and protect here, too!

Daily Care – Every Morning and Every Night

- **Cleanse:** Cleansing your face to remove makeup, dirt and oil helps unclog pores and control breakouts. Never go to bed without removing your makeup.

- **Tone:** A mild toner can remove extra makeup, dirt and grime, minimize appearance of pores, restore pH balance and prepare skin to accept your moisturizer.

- **Moisturize:** Choose a moisturizer designed for your age and specific skin type. Many moisturizers contain vitamins to counter the effects of environmental damage on your skin's surface.

- **Protect:** Use a moisturizer with Sun Protection Factor (SPF) 15 or higher every day, regardless of the season. Continuous direct or indirect exposure to the sun (even through your car's closed window) can cause premature aging of skin, irregular pigmentation like brown spots and potentially, skin cancer. Apply at least 20 minutes before sun exposure and reapply often, especially after perspiring or swimming.

Tips to Improve Your Skin's Appearance

- Eat a balanced diet, low in fat and full of fruits and vegetables.

- Establish a simple daily skincare routine... cleanse, tone, moisturize and protect.

- Protect yourself from the sun's harmful rays, the number one cause of skin damage and wrinkling. Use a sunscreen (minimum SPF 15) on all exposed areas of skin each and every day and consider a daily moisturizer or foundation with sunscreen added.

- Use a sunless tanning product and avoid tanning beds and "laying out."

- Eat a diet rich in antioxidants such as berries, citrus fruits and dark green, leafy vegetables. Antioxidants help skin cells repair and rejuvenate.

- To ensure your vitamin and mineral intake meets the needs of your skin health, dermatologists recommend selenium, Vitamin E, Vitamin C and Vitamin B-Complex to support healthy skin.

- Activities like Yoga, meditation and walking are excellent relaxation techniques for your body. When you are relaxed — mind, body and soul — you are less likely to show furrows and wrinkles on your face. A stress-reducing routine also helps give you life balance.

- Just as dark chocolate may be a simple indulgence in your diet, consider the indulgence of a massage, which increases circulation, promoting healthier-looking skin. In addition to the beauty boost, you may also feel less stressed. For quick stress relief, consider asking your spouse or friend to massage your neck and shoulders.

Exfoliate: Once a week, you should remove dead skin cells to stimulate cell turnover. Consider using a mild (fine-grained) exfoliant to reduce fine lines and reveal healthier, more radiant skin.

Hydrate: Water is the most plentiful substance in the body, accounting for 50-70% of total body weight. Since your body cannot store water, you must constantly replenish it. Drink water and establish a healthy diet rich in antioxidants to promote healthy skin. Moisturize your face and body daily to enhance hydration and skin's moisture.

Beauty Through the Ages

Adapt your skincare regimen to keep up with the changing needs of your skin. As you age, the texture and tone of your skin begins to diminish, so you need to consider how to keep your skin healthy every day. As early as your 20s, your skin begins to lose its thickness. Experts say it continues to lose about 7% of its thickness every 10 years thereafter.

Your skin is also affected by seasonal changes. You may notice dry, flaky skin during winter months and excessive oil in the summer. So, "season" your skin with extra hydration in cold months and oil-free moisturizers in hot, humid times. No matter what the season, cleanse, tone, moisturize and protect every day.

My pink velour sweatsuit

My studded belt from Texas

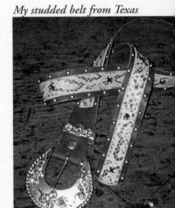

My favorite red pumps

My family

My beaded lamp

Treasured artwork

A Sample Of My Artwork

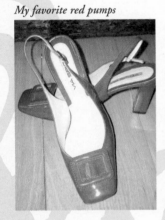

GRIFFEN

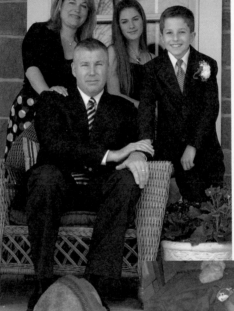

My "babies," Ruby and Rosie

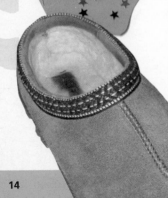

My brown furry Uggs

14

Favorite Things

*A favorite piece
of furniture*

Lisa Klauser

Vice President, Consumer & Customer Solutions ~ Unilever

When Lisa returned her camera loaded with pictures of some her "favorites," she also told us, "My mother is the most impressive woman I know." If you saw Lisa's tribute to her mom in last year's book, you may remember her thank you... "For believing I could do anything I put my mind to... and telling me that when I needed to hear it most."

15

Healthy Skin

As women, we all have a favorite outfit — something we put on our bodies to help us feel special and beautiful. It is just as important to nourish the "outfit we wear every day"... our skin!

Healthy skin is a basic for beauty, and, we're not talking only above the neck. Skin covers every inch of our bodies... so, it's important to care for every inch of our skin. **The good news is...** it's never too late to start taking better care of our skin!

Good, daily, basic skincare should emphasize hydration and moisturizing. To keep skin soft and moist, many dermatologists recommend

Sunless Tan

To give your skin that beautiful "just off the beach" glow and still protect yourself from skin cancers and aging, consider using a self tanning product with an SPF of 15. This will keep you protected from the sun's harmful rays while your sunless tan develops.

The number one contributor to aging skin is harmful rays from the sun. Even moderate exposure to rays can damage skin. The best way to protect your skin is to protect it by wearing sunscreen faithfully, even for everyday exposure. Today's moisturizing products contain sunscreen and daily use gives you double protection... it will keep your skin moisturized AND protect it from further damage.

soaking and sealing. This, they say, is a great way to keep skin from drying out any time of year. Soak skin — whether by taking a shower or a bath in warm water — then immediately seal it with a moisturizer to keep skin soft. When you bathe, use a mild and moisturizing cleansing product. After bathing, gently pat away excess water, then immediately apply moisturizer. Moisturizers that are applied to hydrated skin are more effectively absorbed into the top layer of the skin. A well-balanced moisturizer promotes long-term dry skin healing and provides a more effective barrier against moisture loss.

Whether the moisturizer you use is in the form of an ointment, cream, lotion or gel will depend on your personal preference. The important thing is to find a moisturizer you will want to use at least daily, preferably after your bath or shower, and with a Sun Protection Factor (SPF). Keep a small tube or bottle of a good moisturizer in your purse, pocket or desk so that if your skin feels dry and itchy at any point during the day, you'll have relief close by.

The key to beautiful skin is finding good skincare products that you will enjoy using on a daily basis.

Maintain Balance

The fact is that one of the best ways to keep your skin healthy is to take care of your overall health and well-being. Here are some lifestyle tips to get you started:

- **Get plenty of rest.** There's no question that the general condition of your body, and mind for that matter, is reflected in your skin. While everyone requires a different amount of sleep to feel well-rested, many people complain that they are never rested enough. The average amount of nightly sleep that is required for good health is considered to be approximately 7 – 8 hours.

- **Be gentle with your skin.** Use a nonsoap cleanser and wash only once a day with cleanser. For example, you can wash in the morning with your cleanser and rinse in the evening with tap water alone. Or if you prefer, you can wash in the evening to remove makeup and simply rinse your face gently in the morning. Once or twice a week, it is reasonable to use a mild exfoliant to remove dead skin and promote new cell growth.

- **Have a drink.** Just as our bodies require fluids daily, so does our skin. Be sure to drink plenty of water each day (a minimum of eight glasses).

- **Moisturize your skin on a daily basis.** Many people find that in the dry winter months, it is necessary to moisturize 2 or 3 times a day. Dry skin is uncomfortable and scratching may lead to superficial skin infections, especially when the resulting itch leads to unending scratching. One way to block this vicious cycle is to ensure that your skin is well moisturized. You may never realize how dry your skin really is until you have started to moisturize on a regular basis.

- **Eat well and exercise.** This is not so much specific advice for good skin health, as it is well-established guidance for overall well-being. Try to walk for at least 30 minutes 3 or 4 times a week. Exercise increases circulation that delivers nutrients throughout the body and promotes restful sleep, which allows skin time to rejuvenate. In addition, eat a balanced diet and a variety of foods (see Chapter 5).

> There is no question that if you are in good
> physical shape, your skin will reflect it. If you are rested
> and emotionally whole, your skin will be radiant.

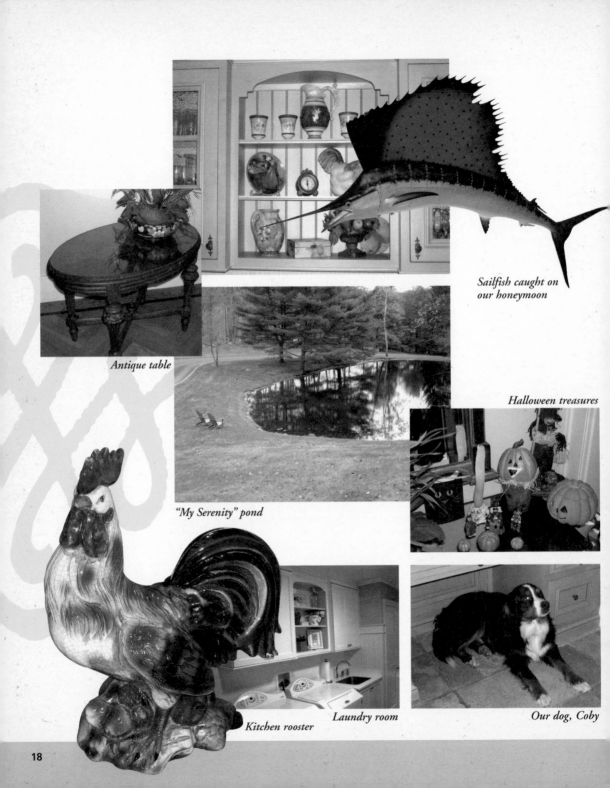

Antique table

Sailfish caught on
our honeymoon

Halloween treasures

"My Serenity" pond

Kitchen rooster

Laundry room

Our dog, Coby

A FEW OF MY
Favorite Things

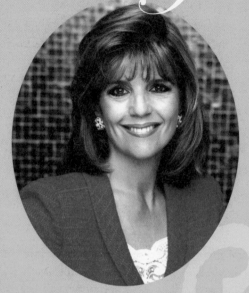

Karen Fondu

President ~ Maybelline/Garnier

Karen loves... Eating out with friends... North Carolina... frozen yogurt... Maui... her favorite book, "God Calling"... favorite singer, Elton John... favorite movie, "Legends of the Fall"... and, she loves Barbie. The most impressive person she's ever met is George Bush, Sr. And, when it comes to favorite makeup, she says, "It's Maybelline New York, of course!"

Favorite Beauty Tips

If one of your favorite things is the process of preparing for a special night out, you should think about extending this favorite into your everyday routine.

Look your best and have fun indulging yourself every day by experimenting with new colors, a new shade of lipstick or gloss or adding a bronzer for extra glow. Try a new hairstyle or a new color. The key is to begin with healthy skin and hair and then to make the most of it for added beauty.

Learn to make the most of your assets!

Let your lips look as fresh as the words that come out of them...

Have fun with lip color. Lips are one of the easiest ways to be adventurous... after all, you can take it off as easily as you put it on.

- Begin with a liner to define the shape of your lips and reduce "feathering" around your lip line. Choose a liner close to your lip's natural color, or choose one that matches the lipcolor.

- Thought you couldn't wear intense colors? Think again. Believe it or not, there's even a red that's right for you. But bold is not your only option... it's also sexy to go nude. Let your mood set the stage. After all, why should all of your moods have to share the same shade?

- Finally, choose a gloss for added shine and radiance.

Have Fun with Cosmetics

Just as an artist starts with a flawless canvas, think of your face as your foundation. Look for products that will play well with your skin type — normal, oily, dry or combination.

Decide How Much Coverage You Want

If you have any blemishes or unevenness, use foundation to give you coverage to even out your complexion. Healthy, unblemished skin doesn't need to be totally covered. Apply face products selectively in areas of uneven skin tone, usually along your nose and cheeks. For a more natural look, use concealer to hide small imperfections and add blush or bronzer to brighten your entire face. If you have oily or combination skin, keep shine under control with a translucent powder.

Add Drama to Your Eyes and Lips

Since eyes are so expressive, you can bring attention to their natural beauty with a simple application of shadow, liner and mascara for lush, full lashes. Or, for evening drama, try a trendy iridescent shadow or layer colors for added effect. Experiment to find what's best for you and what you are comfortable wearing.

Helpful Makeup Tips

Keep cosmetics and applicators (brushes, sponges) clean and bacteria-free. When dirty or worn, replace them. Never share applicators or products with friends or family. Bacteria can easily spread. Replace mascara every 3 months. Most tube and wand mascaras have an antibacterial agent in them that will keep you safe for 2 – 3 months, but the longer you keep the mascara, the more you risk eye infection. If you notice the smell changes or the texture changes, throw it out. If you have an eye infection, replace all of your eye makeup and applicators immediately.

Just as we take care to moisturize and protect our skin, we can't forget our hair.

First, cleanse and protect. Choose a shampoo formulated for your "type." If you have oily skin, you will likely have an oily scalp; same for dry skin and hair. If your hair is color-treated, you'll need a shampoo that won't fade your color. Many of today's products can also add volume to fine, limp hair or provide a boost with added shine. The important thing is to generously shampoo your hair with warm water. Take a few moments to massage your scalp with your fingertips or knuckles. Finish with a conditioner to lock in moisture and protect your hair from environmental influences.

Next, make the most of your hairstyle. We've all seen a gorgeous hairstyle in a magazine and wondered how it would look on us. A good stylist will work with you to achieve the look you want, taking into account the following:

- **Your hair's basic texture.** If your hair is straight and fine, a curly style may not be your best choice. But, you can work with your stylist to learn tricks to boost your hair's volume to achieve the look you desire.

- **How much time and talent do you have?** This is important. Be realistic! If you're typically a "wash-and-go" type, be honest with your stylist about what you're willing and able to do to make a style work.

- **Budget.** Most experts agree that hair requires a trim every 6 – 8 weeks. Figure out what fits realistically into your household budget for haircare. Choose a stylist and a cut that meets your needs.

Finally, have fun with color!

Whether you're interested in just coloring the gray, boosting shine and radiance with an overall color or adding highlights... there are plenty of options. Choose a product that gives you the look you want without sacrificing your hair's health. Permanent, all-over color requires a touch up to cover roots every 6 – 8 weeks. A semi-permanent will fade or wash out in about 24 shampoos. Choose the product that's easiest to work with and best meets your needs.

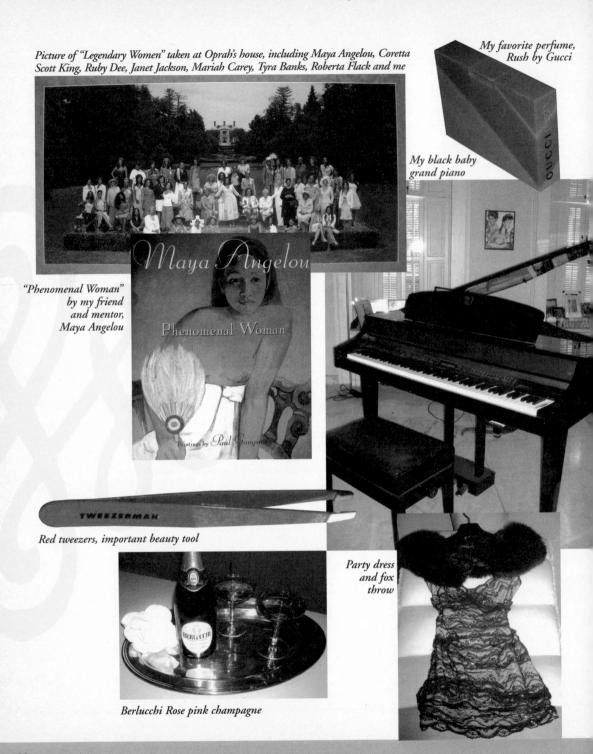

Picture of "Legendary Women" taken at Oprah's house, including Maya Angelou, Coretta Scott King, Ruby Dee, Janet Jackson, Mariah Carey, Tyra Banks, Roberta Flack and me

My favorite perfume, Rush by Gucci

My black baby grand piano

"Phenomenal Woman" by my friend and mentor, Maya Angelou

Maya Angelou

Phenomenal Woman

Paintings by Paul Gauguin

Red tweezers, important beauty tool

TWEEZERMAN

Party dress and fox throw

BERLUCCHI

Berlucchi Rose pink champagne

A FEW OF MY
Favorite Things

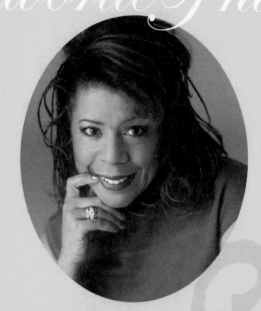

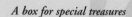

A box for special treasures

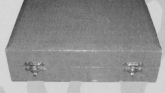

Valerie Simpson

Celebrity Spokeswoman ~ Speaking of Women's Health & Universal Sisters

My red evening shoes and bag,
a birthday gift from Luther Vandross

Grammy award winner, singer, songwriter, wonderful friend, woman of valor, and most importantly to Speaking of Women's Health, Valerie Simpson is a volunteer celebrity spokeswoman who exemplifies our motto, "Be Strong. Be Healthy. Be in Charge."

Healthy Relationships

Our readers have shared with us that one of their favorite things is their friendships. As human beings, relationships with others are one of the most rewarding experiences we have in our lifetimes.

These spiritual, emotional and physical relationships help sustain and fulfill us day-in and day-out and comfort us when we need it. It is a rare gift to meet someone with whom you instantly "connect." More often, relationships develop over time, and require effort on both parts to sustain them. Speaking of Women's Health relationship expert Evelyn Resh, MPH, RN, CNM from Canyon Ranch suggests these tips to healthy, fulfilling friendships:

1. You cannot change how someone else behaves. Each of us can only control our own behaviors, including our responses to what others do and say.

2. Honesty is critically important in all relationships, even when what you have to say is difficult for someone to hear.

3. Humor is an excellent management tool when things become stressful in a relationship.

4. Do your best to maintain compassion at all times toward the other person AND yourself. This will help guide you in many ways.

5. Be willing to look at your own contributions to strife and upset. Relationships are dynamic and it "takes two to tango."

6. Apologizing when you have hurt someone's feelings or done something wrong is very helpful. This can be especially powerful in our relationships with children.

7. Don't extend yourself beyond what is in the best interest of your health. If you lose your health and wellness, it won't serve anyone.

8. Decide what your bottom line is in a situation or relationship, and don't go beyond it.

9. When a relationship involves you giving and never receiving, raise it with the other person. If it doesn't change, let the relationship go.

10. Use pleasure as a matter of measure when evaluating a relationship. You should be able to identify more pleasure than displeasure and if the balance is off, then something is wrong.

When it comes to lasting relationships, laughter truly is the best medicine!

The best relationships are those that don't take themselves too seriously. "Friends who laugh together, stay together!" Having a bad day? Try the Smile Game! You will be surprised at how much happiness you will get out of this. When you are walking down the street or are anywhere around other people, make eye contact with as many people as you can and smile. You'll soon find that smiling is contagious... when someone smiles at you, you can't help but smile in return!

Heart-to-Heart

One common relationship problem is transferring feelings of anger to your spouse or friend when you are really angry at someone else. Who isn't guilty of coming home in a bad mood and losing patience with the kids or spouse because *you* had a bad day at work? Healthy relationships can survive this occasionally, but when it builds and occurs frequently, it can become a much larger problem.

Learn to say "I'm sorry," and more importantly, learn to forgive — one another and yourself.

Don't let resentment and anger build without getting it out in the open. This can only lead to trouble. Find a common ground and work from there to repair the rift.

Take the first step. Mending a broken friendship often requires that one person make the first call.

Don't let days, weeks or even months pass before you address the problem. Or, consider that on some points, it may be best to "agree to disagree" and move on. Who said you have be in step 100% of the time to be friends?

Be the kind of friend you'd like to have.

Set an example for others and chances are they'll return the favor in kind. Send a card for no reason, pick up some flowers and surprise a co-worker, remember to call to ask how the big meeting went or drop by with dinner when a friend has a sick child. Make an effort to be thoughtful and kind, and chances are, others will respond to you.

Live Passionately!

Relationships that involve intimacy and shared passion can be among the most rewarding you'll experience. Finding a lifelong mate is one thing, but sustaining intimacy and passion throughout life requires some effort from both.

- **Take care of your health.** While relationship harmony definitely impacts passion, hormones and health also impact your sex drive. Make sure you are fit for passion.

- **Improve your body image.** Only you know what you need to do to feel good about your body. A positive body image is attractive.

- **Make time for passion.** Set aside quality time for intimacy. Schedule a "date night" and do what makes you both feel special. A romantic dinner by candlelight (see page 86 for recipes for a "night in") or an afternoon movie together may be just the right touch to lead to intimacy.

- **Be generous.** People who think they are not getting enough in a relationship are often not giving enough.

- **Honor the sexual needs of the relationship.** Monogamy, fidelity, sexual sensitivity, respect, generosity and compassion go hand-in-hand in healthy relationships.

- **Have fun with your partner on a regular basis.** Share the good times with each other. Mutual fun is the shortest route to passion.

- **Discover your passion.** Libido means life energy. A passion for life translates into passion in your relationship.

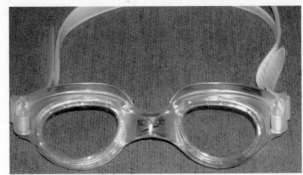

Goggles – I LOVE to swim

My white adirondack chairs

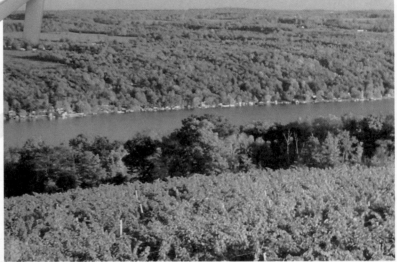

My great, great-grandmother's diamond and sapphire ring

My favorite place to go – Keuka Lake, New York

Family photo

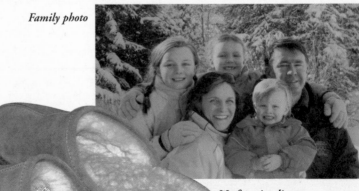

My favorite slippers

A FEW OF MY
Favorite Things

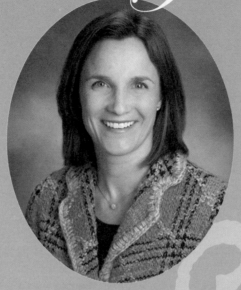

Kim Miller

Vice President, Morning Foods Marketing ~ Kellogg's

We think Kim's "favorites" show her love of family and her sense of generational respect... from her great, great-grandmother's ring to her daughter's fabulous handmade invitation.

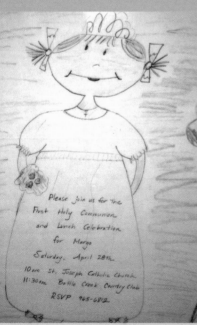

The invitation my daughter Margo made for her 1st Communion

Healthy Eating

Everyone has a favorite holiday, favorite season or a favorite family gathering. Think of your favorites.

Chances are, each occasion or get-together also has a favorite food! In fact, we've filled this book with some of our favorite recipes. Since we began Speaking of Women's Health, we've focused much of our education and motivation on the topic of maintaining a healthy diet, full of fruits and vegetables and low in fat. In fact, you may see it as a golden thread throughout this book. What you eat does have an effect on your health. It is one thing about your health that you can change this very minute! Here's how...

Variety

Perhaps you've noticed that the days of just 4 basic food groups — dairy, meat, vegetables and fruit — are long gone. A healthy diet includes the basics of leafy greens, brightly-colored fruits and berries, low-fat dairy and lean meats and fish. Today we know that there is a delicious range of options that will enhance the basics. These include whole grains, nuts, legumes (beans) and even plant oils, such as olive oil.

The new food pyramid outlines various foods that, if eaten in the right quantities, form the foundation of a healthy diet. No single food provides all of the nutrients your body needs, so eating a variety of foods within each group ensures that you get the necessary nutrients and other substances that promote good health. For example, some healthy meat choices include lean beef, organic chicken and wild salmon, loaded with heart-healthy Omega-3 fatty acids. The fruits and vegetables category could include a leafy green chopped salad with tomatoes, carrots and cucumber. Add a little crushed flax seed, garbanzo beans and top with fresh berries and now you're talking variety! For variety in the grain category, consider whole grain cereals, brown rice and pastas and whole wheat breads. To get your calcium, a good start is from non-fat Vitamin D-fortified milk, low-fat yogurt and a variety of low-fat cheeses.

> According to nutritionist David Meinz, as adults, we need 30 grams of fiber daily. Most Americans only get about 10 grams. Adding fiber to your diet can help control cholesterol, speed the passage of waste through your system, thus decreasing the amount of toxins absorbed and helps your body regulate blood sugar, important for the prevention of diabetes.

Low Fat

Choose a diet that provides no more than 30% of total calories from total fat, and no more than 10% from saturated fat. Saturated fat raises blood cholesterol more than other forms of fat. The fats from meat, milk and milk products are the main sources of saturated fats in most diets. Vegetable oils supply smaller amounts of saturated fat. Partially hydrogenated vegetable oils, known as trans-fatty acids, should be avoided or limited.

Powerful Superfoods

While there's no such thing as a "miracle food," there are certain foods that can help you maintain good health. If you aren't eating these foods already, you don't know what you're missing.

Broccoli – For Vitamin C, fiber, beta carotene and folate.
Toss broccoli florets and chopped stems into your next omelet.

Nuts and Seeds – For fiber, vitamins and minerals.
Sprinkle nuts for extra crunch in your salads, cereal or yogurt.

Soybeans and Soy Products – For B Vitamins, isoflavones and fiber.
Try vanilla or chocolate-flavored, low-calorie soy milk in your next bowl of cereal.

Beans and Legumes – For folate and fiber.
Use beans in place of meat in your favorite chili recipe.

Sweet Potatoes – For Vitamins A and C, beta carotene, potassium and fiber.
Try adding non-fat milk or orange juice to mashed sweet potatoes.

Salmon, Tuna, Rainbow Trout – For Omega-3 fatty acids and unsaturated fats.
At your next barbeque, throw some fish on the grill.

Spinach, Kale, Swiss Chard – For Vitamins A, C, beta carotene, calcium, folate and fiber.
Fill your next lasagna with these leafy greens.

Oranges – For Vitamin C, folate and fiber.
Next time you need to deglaze your sauté pan, try orange juice.

Tomatoes – For lycopene, Vitamin C and potassium.
Puree tomatoes with other vegetables and spices for a delicious cold soup.

Whole Grains and Whole Grain Breads and Cereals – For B Vitamins and fiber.
Add whole grains, like cooked brown rice to ground meat for extra body.

Blueberries – For Vitamins A and C, potassium, folate, fiber and antioxidants.
Frozen blueberries are great to keep on hand for smoothies, pancakes and desserts.

Water – Drink up!

It is essential that you refresh your body with plenty of water to replenish body fluids, rid your body of illness-producing toxins and help you maintain a healthy weight. Women who are physically active, live in warm environments, or who are pregnant or breast feeding should increase their intake of fluids.

Occasional Indulgences

The secret to healthy eating is moderation, in other words portion control. So, we're giving you permission, in fact we're encouraging you to have an occasional small indulgence. Try our brownie recipe (see page 63) but cut the portion in half. Eat it slowly and savor each bite. And, don't forget... dark chocolate is a potent antioxidant. Eaten in moderation, and in combination with a healthy diet as described in this chapter, dark chocolate may even help lower cholesterol and blood pressure.

A tree named "Fred," given to my mom about 20 years ago. Here is a picture of "Fred" with Caroline.

My daughters' artwork. I frame and decorate my house with my favorites.

sisters

CHAT NOIR

I love making gingerbread people pancakes with my daughters

A ceramic pig named Maximillian, a gift from my husband

A FEW OF MY
Favorite Things

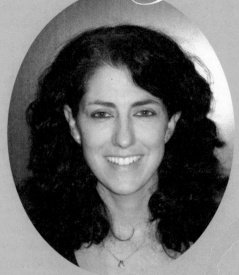

Sarah Egan

Director, One A Day Franchise & Children's Vitamins ~ Bayer

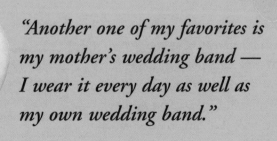

"Another one of my favorites is my mother's wedding band — I wear it every day as well as my own wedding band."

Supplement Your Health

If one of your favorite things is having the confidence that you are giving your body the vitamins and nutrients it needs, you will find this chapter very helpful.

Our panel of experts agree that eating a healthy diet, exercising and reducing the stress in your life will help you build a stronger immune system. However, even if you ate the "perfect" diet every day, your body may not get all it needs. That is why so many nutrition and medical experts suggest adding a supplement.

There are specific vitamins and minerals that can help us at different stages of our lives. Begin with your pharmacist or health care professional for recommendations on which supplements will best support your overall health and ensure they won't interfere or react with any medications or herbal supplements you may take.

Recently-published studies suggest that Vitamin D may help prevent breast cancer. Vitamin D, also known as the sunshine vitamin because our bodies produce it from sunlight, is also valuable because it helps our bodies absorb calcium, essential for bone health.

Dietary supplements will help improve your health regardless of what you eat, but taken in combination with a well-rounded diet, your health may achieve even higher levels.

What are Vitamins and Minerals?

Vitamins are sometimes referred to as the "spark plugs" of our human machine. They are required to do many things and their excess or depletion can lead to acute and chronic disease. Vitamins are an essential part of the body's metabolic processes, playing a vital role in its enzyme systems.

Minerals such as calcium, iron, zinc and potassium are necessary to help build strong bones, transmit nerve impulses, make hormones and maintain a normal heart beat.

Because the body is unable to manufacture most vitamins by itself, we need to ingest them from outside sources. Ideally, we should obtain these vitamins from consuming a healthy diet consisting of a wide variety of foods. Often, however, our diets are not adequate and, in some cases, our bodies are not able to consume the recommended daily amounts of vitamins and minerals from food alone.

What Should Your Daily Supplement Include?

Let's take a look at what the experts recommend for each stage of a healthy woman's life. As you age and your body becomes less efficient at processing nutrients, your needs for a multivitamin may change. Talk to your pharmacist or health care professional for advice based on your age, dietary habits and any medical conditions you may have.

Calcium. As you'll read in Chapter 19, calcium is essential for building and maintaining strong bones, our bodies' framework. To assure that calcium is absorbed by your body, it is necessary to include Vitamin D and magnesium. Many women find it difficult to get adequate amounts from diet alone, so a supplement may be recommended. But, if you take a supplement, remember that your body can only absorb so much calcium at a time... so, take it in split doses both morning and night, instead of all at once.

Iron. Women and adolescents of menstruating age are advised to maintain adequate levels of iron to help build and maintain red blood cells that carry oxygen to tissues.

Zinc. Zinc supports our body's normal growth and development throughout childhood and adolescence, as well as helping to maintain a healthy immune system and is necessary for wound healing.

Potassium. This mineral is essential because it helps regulate blood pressure, is used in muscle contraction and helps convert blood sugar into energy.

Selenium. This mineral has antioxidant properties that, according to some studies, may decrease the death rate from lung, colorectal and prostate cancers and may promote heart health.

Beta Carotene. Confused about Vitamin A and beta carotene? Remember the saying that all robins are birds, but all birds are not robins? Same idea. All beta carotenes are A Vitamins, but all A Vitamins are not beta carotenes. You need Vitamin A and beta carotene. Beta carotene is an antioxidant and helps the body fight cancer by attacking destructive free radicals. Research indicates that beta carotene might also protect against cardiovascular disease and memory loss, but more studies are needed to confirm the association.

Vitamin A. Vitamin A plays an important role in vision, bone growth, reproduction, cell division and cell differentiation and helps regulate the immune system.

Vitamin C. This antioxidant helps hold body cells together and strengthens walls of blood vessels, helps in healing wounds, helps to build bones and teeth and aids in the absorption of iron.

Vitamin E. Helps keep red blood cells intact. This antioxidant protects Vitamin A and essential fatty acids from oxidation. It also helps maintain normal muscle metabolism. Recent studies suggest that a Vitamin E-rich diet can help protect some people against Alzheimer's disease.

The B Vitamins. The Bs, including folic acid, help our body's cells obtain energy from food. They help keep nerves in healthy condition and promote good appetite and digestion. They also promote healthy skin, eyes, clear vision and are needed to build healthy red blood cells. And, the B Vitamins are essential for normal development during pregnancy.

Folic Acid. New research shows that folic acid may cut the risk of heart disease and stroke by lowering the body's homocystine levels. Women who are pregnant are advised to increase their daily intake of folic acid. Talk to your physician or health care provider.

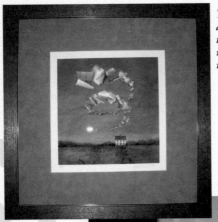

This piece of art is a beacon to encourage me to write more

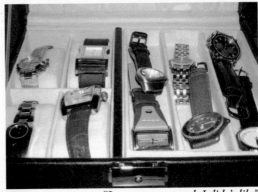

"I never met a watch I didn't like"

My babies are Dante (11) and Lori (12). They are my "snugglebugs."

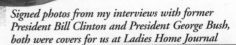

A piece of pottery made by a very close friend. I love its classic shape and bold, rich, almost majestic colors.

My special pillow

Signed photos from my interviews with former President Bill Clinton and President George Bush, both were covers for us at Ladies Home Journal

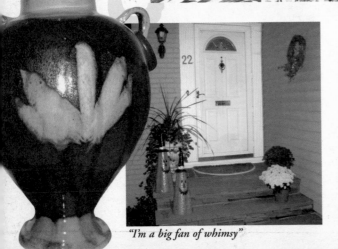

"I'm a big fan of whimsy"

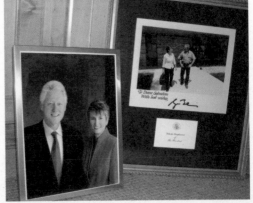

A FEW OF MY
Favorite Things

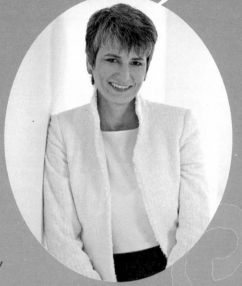

Favorite books – part of our cover story

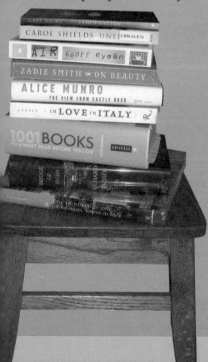

Diane Salvatore

Editor-in-Chief ~ Ladies Home Journal

Diane wrote, "Thanks so much for inviting me to be in the 'Favorite Things' book. It was indeed a very delicious exercise!"

Speaking of Women's Health wants to thank Diane for giving us such a great photo that it could be part of "our cover."

Step It Up~Be Active

Most of us remember the days when our favorite things included running, exploring, jumping, laughing — all fun activities that involved movement.

Finding ways to incorporate just 30 minutes of "exercise" into each day will help you enjoy the benefits of weight control and better health, improved self-esteem and balance — physically, emotionally and even spiritually.

For all that we know about the benefits of physical activity, many women (roughly 60%) still do not engage in activity. If you're one of them... get moving!

If you were to exercise for about 30 minutes most days, you could:

- Lower your cholesterol and blood pressure levels
- Improve your sleep
- Increase oxygen to the brain and improve memory
- Make your bones stronger and improve posture
- Burn stored body fat to help you lose weight
- Reduce stress and tension
- Increase energy
- Protect your body from injury and disease
- Slow the aging process
- Boost self-confidence

For most women, a combination of the 3 types of exercise are important to consider.

Weight-Bearing Activity. Weight-bearing exercise improves muscle strength and builds bones because your body bears its own weight. The easiest weight-bearing activity is walking — others include carrying groceries, dancing, bowling, golfing (carry your own bag) and even gardening. If you belong to a gym, use the machines to work all major muscle groups. Do not work the same groups on back–to–back days. Don't belong to a gym? Don't own hand weights yet? Get started today. Grab a can of soup in each hand and start lifting.

Aerobic Activity. Aerobic activity is any exercise that uses large muscle groups and gets the heart and lungs working and pumping. Examples are bicycling, swimming, jogging or brisk walking, dancing, playing volleyball, tennis, racquetball, soccer, softball, basketball or skating. Aerobic exercise helps strengthen your heart muscles to keep them working effectively. How about a game of tag with your kids, grandkids or other young people in your life?

Stretching Activity. Stretching is essential for maintaining muscle health and increased flexibility. If you're one of many women with chronic back pain, begin and end each day with gentle stretching to loosen your back muscles. Yoga is a great activity that focuses on balance, breathing, strength building and flexibility. It combines deep breathing, relaxation and mindful focus while you stretch and balance in simple, easy postures. Look for beginner's videos to follow or seek a class in your neighborhood or near work.

Even a Little Time is On Your Side

Small steps equal big rewards... start with 10 minutes a day, and make it fun! With a bit of creativity you can make time for exercise!

- Set the alarm early on Monday morning and start the week with a walk.

- Meet your child's bus and walk home... the long way! Take turns carrying the backpack and you'll both build strong bones!

- Invite other parents to join you in circling the soccer field or walking the halls at school during basketball practice.

- Keep some 5-pound hand weights in your desk and car so you can take advantage of downtime to build arm strength.

- Enjoy a Yoga video or DVD or, join a class at the Y or local church or Yoga studio.

- Shorten your lunch and take a walk with co-workers. Have a meeting? Ask the participant to go for a walk and talk, instead of sitting at a desk or table... then send a quick e-mail to recap the discussion and next steps.

- Pick a night and go dancing! Salsa dance or boot scoot to healthier bones!

- Look for ways to incorporate weight-bearing exercise into your housecleaning routine... carrying laundry up and down stairs, bringing groceries into the house and bending to load and unload the dishwasher.

- Make errand day, activity day! Park in one central location and walk to the drycleaner, video store and library.

- After dinner, ask the kids to clean up while you and your spouse, or neighbor, go for a walk.

- Start your morning off with 10 minutes of gentle stretching to energize and wake your body.

- Take a walk after your religious services to reflect on the day's messages.

- Enjoy your favorite TV program, the guilt-free way. Do some leg lifts and stretching during the commercial breaks.

- Need to get some shopping done? Put on your walking shoes and go for it! Challenge yourself to move throughout the store and walk each aisle for added activity.

KEY LEARNING...
More than 50% of women over the age of 50 will suffer a broken bone. Maintaining your balance will help you avoid falls that may cause breaks. Developing your flexibility will help you maintain balance.

Comfort is very important for activity. Choose lightweight clothing that breathes and allows moisture to evaporate or materials that actually wick away moisture from your skin. Affordable exercise clothing can be found almost anywhere, and today's styles are even fashionable enough to wear outside of the gym. Be sure your clothing does not restrict movement or cause discomfort. Also, wear a supportive bra that fits properly to relieve breast discomfort.

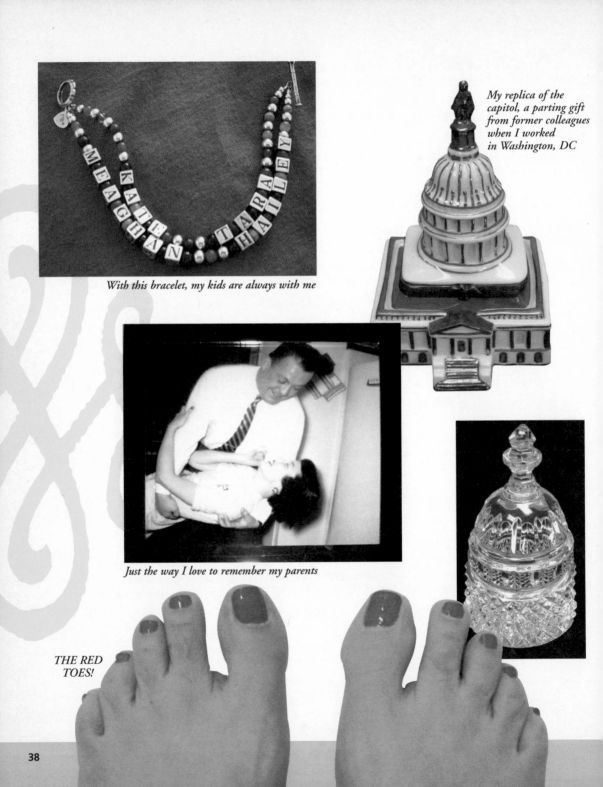

With this bracelet, my kids are always with me

My replica of the capitol, a parting gift from former colleagues when I worked in Washington, DC

Just the way I love to remember my parents

THE RED TOES!

A FEW OF MY
Favorite Things

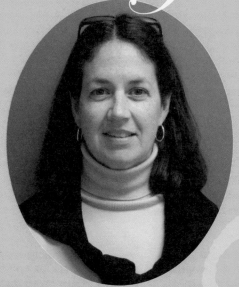

Kelly Downey

Director of Shopper Marketing ~ Unilever

"Pedicures and red toes! My one indulgence! And my flip flops... I would wear them in the winter if my kids didn't see that as a tactic endorsement as permission to do the same. (Also works well showing off red toes!)"

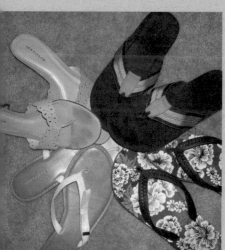

"Year-round" footwear

Find Your Healthy Weight

Achieving and maintaining your healthy weight can mean the
difference between enjoying your favorite activities or
enduring chronic pain, illness and depression.

Obesity is the number one health risk facing women in America today. Think those extra pounds are no big deal? Obesity is defined as having a Body Mass Index (BMI) of 30 or above (log on to www.speakingofwomenshealth.com to calculate your BMI and target your healthy weight). Obesity is responsible for most cases of type 2 diabetes. Diabetes is the number one cause of heart disease and heart disease is the number one killer of women in America.

The fact is, while many diet programs may claim differently, there is only one way to lose weight. Decrease the amount of calories your body stores. This means either eat fewer calories OR burn more. A combination of the two is the best choice.

For many women on-the-go, impulse eating choices are often part of the problem. Our Speaking of Women's Health experts agree that planning to eat healthy is an important part of making it happen.

- On the weekend, think through the week's activities. Sit down with the family calendar and plan at least 4 dinners. This is a great time to make your grocery list also. Post the menus on the refrigerator and enlist the help of the entire family to make it happen.

- Pre-packaged, snack-sized portions of carrots, cheese, fruits and bite-sized veggies are available. Convenient 100-calorie packages of cookies and snacks are great to keep on hand. Make them easy to reach for... keep plenty on hand and in an obvious place.

- Consider packing a cooler with healthy snacks and cold drinks to help curb hunger throughout the day's activities. Keep healthy snacks on hand at the office also. If your office is celebrating something with cake, don't miss out on the fun. If you must indulge, have a few bites instead of the whole piece.

- Many women tell us that once they adapt to healthier eating... they actually save money! The key is keeping your kitchen stocked with ready-to-eat healthy choices for the entire family and keeping healthy snacks accessible.

Don't Forget the Second Part of the Equation... Physical Activity

One reason that so many people are overweight today compared with 50 years ago is the prevalence of technology in our lives. We drive from the garage to the office. We drive to the market and often the bus stop or mailbox. We turn on the TV or computer to reach out to the world and even our neighbors. 50 years ago, Americans spent more time walking in the course of a given day. Why? Because, our communities encouraged parking in one central location and walking to multiple destinations.

A healthy lifestyle requires daily physical activity. How can you build exercise into your routine? It's not as difficult as you may think.

- Take a note from our healthy eating suggestions and prepare meals and menus ahead of time. When you get home from the office, pop the casserole into the oven, set the timer for 45 minutes, THEN spend that time moving your body! Meet your neighbor or spouse and walk while you catch up on the day. Grab the family dog and take a quick hike. Put the kids in the stroller and go for a spin. Older kids may enjoy a bike ride after school. You'll arrive home energized for the evening activities.

- Encourage other parents at your child's practices and rehearsals to move with you. Take advantage of the time you normally spend waiting and get moving!

- Set aside ME time to focus on your own health and well-being. This is not being selfish... this is being proactive. You need to be healthy and emotionally balanced to do your best every day for yourself and those you love and care for!

Be Good to Your Body, Be Good to the Earth

Eat more locally-grown fruits and vegetables. Your food will be fresher, and it will take less energy to get the food from the ground to your table. This will naturally increase the amount of fruits and vegetables you eat. Think of it as your own PSP – Personal Sustainability Plan (a concept originally developed to help Wal-Mart Associates live healthier)!

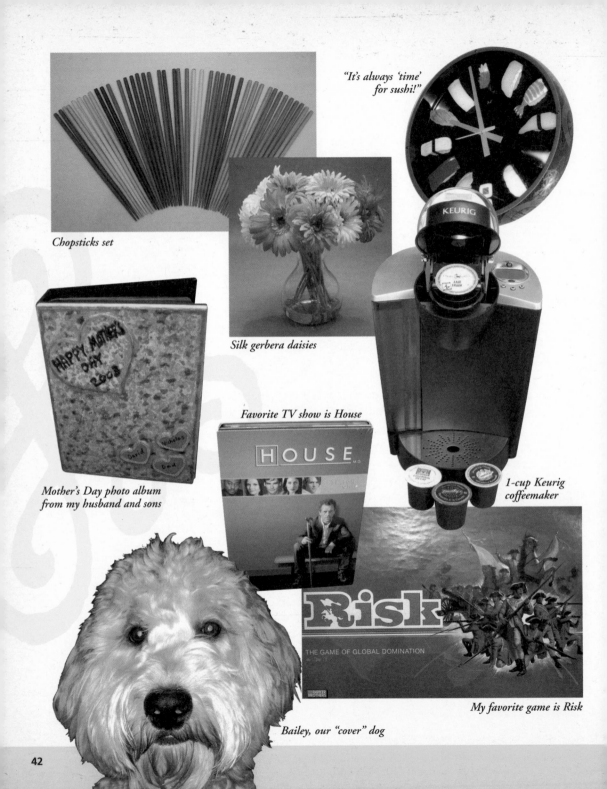

Chopsticks set

"It's always 'time' for sushi!"

Silk gerbera daisies

Mother's Day photo album from my husband and sons

HAPPY MOTHER'S DAY 2008

Favorite TV show is House

1-cup Keurig coffeemaker

Bailey, our "cover" dog

My favorite game is Risk

A FEW OF MY
Favorite Things

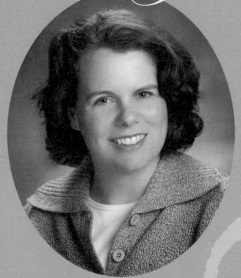

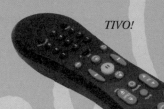

TIVO!

Jane Ghosh

Director of Marketing ~ Kellogg's

Jane says her favorite place to go regularly is Chicago and her favorite place she's ever been is Koh Samui, Thailand. We're guessing she loves to read The New Yorker, Harper's and The Atlantic while she's on the plane.

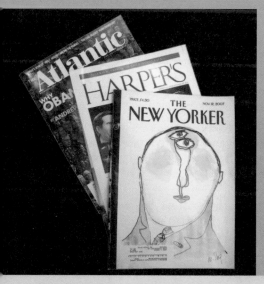

Heart Health & Cholesterol

If one of your favorite things is having people say about you, "She has a really **good** heart," you're on the right track to being not only a **good** person, but a **healthy** person.

Having a good heart and a healthy heart should both be priorities in your life (actually, studies show that being kind and having a positive outlook can be helpful to avoid heart attacks).

Unfortunately, many people still believe that heart disease is primarily a men's health problem. Actually, heart disease is the number one killer of women. 37% of women in America die of heart disease, and if you include stroke, that number jumps to 50%. **The good news is...** heart disease is largely preventable and treatable.

While there are many different forms of heart disease, the most common is a narrowing or blockage of the coronary arteries, the blood vessels that supply blood to the heart itself. This is called coronary artery disease (CAD) and happens slowly over time. It is the major reason people have heart attacks.

Other kinds of heart problems may happen to the valves in the heart, or the heart may not pump well and cause heart failure. There are specific tests to determine your risk. Visit **www.speakingofwomenshealth.com** for more information.

You can help reduce your risk of heart disease by taking steps to control factors that put you at greater risk:

- **Control your blood pressure.** Have it checked regularly. An ideal blood pressure is 120/80. It's important to know your numbers and have your pressure checked regularly. Many people can maintain or lower their blood pressure through diet and exercise. For others, medication is essential. Talk to your health care provider. If medication is prescribed, never, ever skip a dose unless specifically directed to do so by your health care provider.

- **Don't smoke.** Smoking is the number one risk factor for heart disease because it increases blood pressure, decreases exercise tolerance and increases the tendency for blood to clot. Smoking also increases the risk of recurrent coronary heart disease after bypass surgery. If you smoke... **Stop Today!** There are excellent over-the-counter smoking cessation resources as well as online support groups.

- **Get enough exercise.** Exercise builds the muscles that move blood and oxygen throughout your body. See Chapter 7 for more information.

- **Maintain a healthy cholesterol profile.** Have your cholesterol tested.

How often should I have my cholesterol checked?

All adults age 20 or older should have a fasting lipoprotein profile — which measures total cholesterol, LDL (bad) cholesterol, HDL (good) cholesterol and triglycerides — once every 5 years, unless your doctor recommends it more frequently.

A heart-healthy "diet" isn't just what you eat... it's your healthy-heart action plan. Eating a heart-healthy diet and maintaining a good exercise program should be a daily habit to keep your cholesterol profile where it should be for a long and healthy life.

Daily exercise and a few simple changes in your diet can help you achieve optimal blood cholesterol levels and protect your heart.

A few simple diet changes:

- Switch to very low-fat or fat-free dairy products.
- Minimize the amount of fat you add to foods. Choose fat-free salad dressings, mayonnaise, sour cream, cream cheese and heart-healthy buttery spreads.
- Season steamed vegetables with spices and herbs.
- Bake, boil, grill or broil foods. If you must fry, spray the pan with a non-stick cooking spray or choose a heart-healthy buttery spread.
- Use liquid vegetable oils rather than solid vegetable shortening. Choose olive, canola or sunflower oils.

A few healthy choices each day can add up to many years of health and well-being.

Surviving a Heart Attack

First, know the symptoms. These often differ for women and may include:

- A feeling of breathlessness or anxiety
- Flu-like symptoms — nausea, clamminess
- Pain in the upper back, neck, shoulders or jaw
- Unexplained, excessive fatigue and difficulty sleeping

Heart Attack Action Plan

If you've already had a heart attack or your doctor has told you that you are at high risk for having a heart attack, be prepared. If you experience symptoms:

- **CALL 9-1-1**
- While you wait for the ambulance to arrive, chew one regular tablet of aspirin (do not take the aspirin if you are allergic to aspirin)
- Put a nitroglycerin tablet under your tongue
- Have the address of the nearest hospital with emergency cardiac care facilities readily available
- Have your resting ECG available
- Keep a list of medications you are taking and a list of your allergies

My musical statues

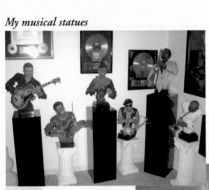

My awards corner

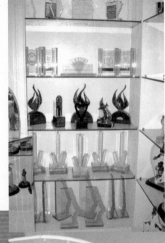

My baby grand piano

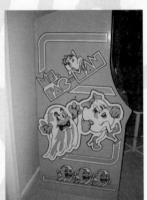

My Pac-Man arcade game –
I can play all night

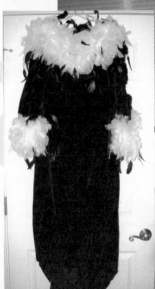

My favorite gown

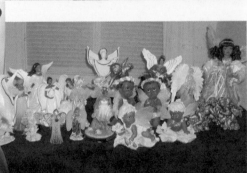

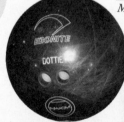

My bowling balls

My angels keep watch over me

A FEW OF MY
Favorite Things

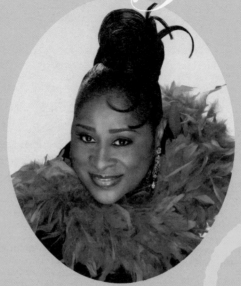

Dottie Peoples

Celebrity Spokeswoman ~ Speaking of Women's Health & Universal Sisters

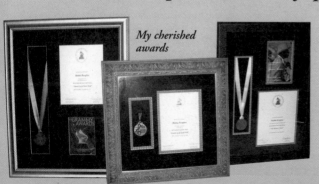

My cherished awards

Known as the "Songbird of the South," our Queen of Gospel, Miss Dottie Peoples is a celebrity spokeswoman for Speaking of Women's Health. It is clear from her favorite photos that her music and her spirituality guide her and her millions of fans across the world.

Stroke –
Know The Facts

*If one of your favorite things is living life to its fullest...
then keep this information top of mind.*

Despite gains in awareness, a 2003 American Heart Association study of more than 1,000 women revealed that a mere 13% of women in America believe that stroke and heart disease are the greatest health threat to women. This statistic reveals the lack of knowledge and understanding a majority of women have for their most serious health threat.

Like most people, you may think heart disease and stroke are a distant second to cancer as a cause of death among women. And like most people, you'd be dangerously wrong.

In reality, heart attack, stroke and related cardiovascular diseases are responsible for almost twice as many deaths among women as all forms of cancer combined.

Of the 700,000 Americans who have a stroke each year, 39% of those who die are men and 61% are women according to the National Stroke Association.

Think and Act FAST!

Every minute counts for stroke patients and acting F.A.S.T. can lead patients to the stroke treatments they desperately need. The most effective stroke treatments are only available if the stroke is recognized and diagnosed within the first 3 hours of the first symptoms.

Use the following tool to help you recognize stroke symptoms and act F.A.S.T.

FACE	Ask the person to smile. Does one side of the face droop?
ARMS	Ask the person to raise both arms. Does one arm drift downward?
SPEECH	Ask the person to repeat a simple sentence. Are the words slurred? Can he/she repeat the sentence correctly?
TIME & TPA	If the person shows any of these symptoms, time is critical. **Call 9-1-1.** Brain cells are dying. When given within 3 hours of the onset of symptoms, a clot-dissolving drug known as TPA has been proven to reduce the amount of damage due to heart attack or significantly reduce the effects of stroke and reduce permanent disability. TPA can save lives... but, time is critical. If someone is showing signs of a stroke, seek medical attention immediately.

A stroke is also known as a "brain attack" because similarly to a heart attack, in a stroke, blood flow is cut off due to a blockage in the arteries leading to the brain. It may also be due to a brain bleed, which may be caused by an aneurysm that causes a vessel to burst. Common risk factors are divided into 2 categories — those you can and those you cannot control.

Risks that can be controlled with medical treatment and lifestyle changes:

- High blood pressure
- Diabetes
- Cigarette smoking
- Incidence of TIA (mini-strokes)
- High blood cholesterol
- Obesity
- Heart disease

Risks that you cannot control:

- Aging
- Male gender
- Race
- Family history of stroke

Action steps to reduce your risk of stroke:

- Get an annual physical including blood pressure and cholesterol checks
- Maintain a healthy diet
- Be aware of your family history
- Maintain a healthy weight for your body type
- Quit smoking
- Exercise
- Manage your blood sugar levels, if diabetic
- Take your medications as directed

Symptoms of Stroke

Like a heart attack, symptoms of stroke may differ in women than from men.

Common stroke symptoms seen in both men and women:

- Sudden numbness or weakness of face, arm or leg, especially on one side of the body
- Sudden confusion, trouble speaking or understanding
- Sudden trouble seeing in one or both eyes
- Sudden trouble walking, dizziness, loss of balance or coordination
- Sudden severe headache with no known cause

Women may report unique stroke symptoms:

- Sudden face and limb pain
- Sudden hiccups
- Sudden nausea
- Sudden general weakness
- Sudden chest pain
- Sudden shortness of breath
- Sudden palpitations

What is a "mini-stroke?"

A "mini-stroke," also called a transient ischemic attack (TIA), happens when, for a short time, less blood than normal gets to the brain. You may have some signs of stroke or you may not notice any signs. A "mini-stroke" may last from a few minutes up to a day. Many people do not even know they have had a stroke. A "mini-stroke" can be a sign of a full stroke to come. If you think you are having a "mini-stroke," CALL 9-1-1.

Family photos

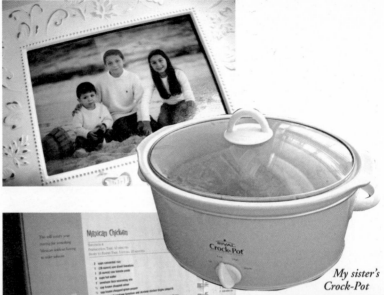

My camera

*My sister's
Crock-Pot*

My gold earrings

A favorite recipe

Dancing shoes

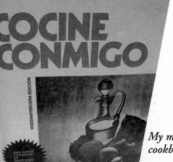

*My mother's
cookbook*

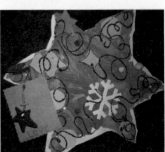

My kids' art projects

A FEW OF MY
Favorite Things

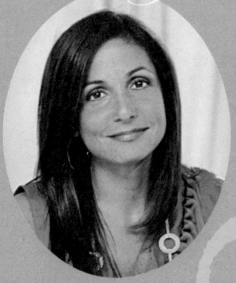

Johanna Buchholtz

Editor-in-Chief, "Siempre Mujer" ~ Meredith

I love summertime, the color gold and I love dancing, (especially salsa and the merengue) and I love entertaining my friends and cooking for them. I love the Spanish singer and composer Alejandro Sanz. I love the sea and water in general, especially the beach at sunset... and oh yes, I especially love my lipstick!

Diabetes Prevention & Management

Many of our favorite possessions are handed down from previous generations. These are treasures that comfort us physically and emotionally.

However, there are other things that are passed down through generations that are not favorites. If your parents or grandparents have or had diabetes, your risk of developing it is greatly increased. While there are some things, like heredity, that we cannot control... there are several risk factors for diabetes that we can control. **"Be Strong. Be Healthy. Be in Charge."** Know your risk factors and take action.

Risk factors you can control

- **Being overweight or obese.** This means having a body mass index (BMI) of 25 or more.
- **High blood pressure.** Having a blood pressure higher than the recommended 120/80 is a risk factor that can be controlled through lifestyle changes, including a healthy diet and daily physical activity. Often, medication is required.
- **Poor cholesterol profile.** This means HDL cholesterol ("good" cholesterol) levels of 35 or lower and/or triglyceride levels of 250 or higher.
- **Inactivity.** Living a sedentary lifestyle (not exercising).

Risk factors you cannot control

- **Heredity.** Having a parent or sibling with type 2 diabetes.
- **Ethnicity.** Being of African American, American Indian/Alaskan Native, Asian/Pacific Islander or Hispanic/Latino.
- **Gestational diabetes.** Having had at least one baby weighing more than 9 pounds at birth.
- **Age.** Approximately 18.4% of Americans over age 65 have type 2 diabetes.
- **Pre-diabetes.** Pre-diabetes means you have blood glucose levels higher than normal, but not high enough to be diagnosed with diabetes. **The good news is...** progression from pre-diabetes to diabetes is not inevitable. Lifestyle changes including modest weight loss and daily exercise can prevent or delay the onset of type 2 diabetes.

Take charge today to prevent the complications of diabetes and to get the most out of life every day! The National Institutes of Health recommends that anyone 45 years old or older should consider getting tested for diabetes. If you are 45 or older and overweight or obese, it is strongly recommended that you get tested regardless of additional risk factors.

When it comes to diabetes, it's time to take charge and stop the epidemic. According to the American Diabetes Association, an estimated 9.3 million women (8.7% of all women) over the age of 20 in the United States have diabetes, and one-third of them remain undiagnosed. The prevalence of diabetes is at least 2–4 times higher among African American, Hispanic/Latino, American Indian and Asian/Pacific Islander women than among white women. The risk for diabetes also increases with age. Because of the increasing lifespan of women and the rapid growth of minority populations, the number of women in the United States at high risk for diabetes and its complications is increasing.

Knowledge is Power...
Learn the Facts

Type 2 diabetes accounts for 90 to 95% of all diabetes cases in America. Unlike type 1 diabetes, where destruction of the pancreas reduces and eventually stops the supply of the hormone insulin, most people with type 2 diabetes are still able to produce insulin at diagnosis. However, the insulin they produce is unable to perform its primary job, which is helping the body's cells use glucose for energy.

If glucose can't be absorbed by the cells, it builds up in the bloodstream instead, and high blood sugar is the result. Over time, the high blood glucose levels from uncontrolled diabetes can cause serious long-term health problems with virtually every system in your body. An early diagnosis is important to prevent some of the other, more serious complications of diabetes, which include heart disease, high blood pressure, nerve damage and kidney failure.

If you have diabetes, consistent eating habits can help you control your blood sugar levels. Every day, try to eat about the same amount of food at about the same time. Include a variety of foods to help meet your nutritional goals. Your dietitian can help you plan a program that meets these guidelines:

NUTRIENT	AIM FOR
Carbohydrates	45 – 65% of daily calories
Protein	15 – 20% of daily calories
Fats	20 – 35% of daily calories
Exercise	Aerobic, weight-bearing and flexibility. Aim for 10 minutes of each type per day.

The good news is... in many cases, type 2 diabetes can be adequately controlled through a combination of proper nutrition and exercise. What can you do to prevent or treat diabetes?

Choose a diet that emphasizes vegetables, fruits and whole grains. Rather than a restrictive diabetes diet, it's a healthy-eating plan that's naturally rich in nutrients and low in fat and calories. In fact, it's the best eating plan for anyone who wants to manage his or her weight by adopting healthier eating habits.

Avoid overeating. Eat 4 – 5 small meals throughout the day before you feel hungry rather than eating 3 large ones.

Exercise daily. Every bit of activity is important. Look for ways to increase your activity levels gradually. Park farther from the entrance to the store. Take a walk around the block after eating or at lunchtime before returning to work. Walk around the field at your child's soccer game (invite other parents to join you for fun).

Talk to your health care professionals. Diabetes is a disease that requires a team approach. You've got to take charge to do your part... that is make the needed lifestyle changes and actively communicate with your health care providers what is happening with your body. This is the best way for your team to make the right decisions regarding your long-term health.

Kids & Teens
Children and adolescents are increasingly at risk for type 2 diabetes due to growing childhood weight problems and sedentary lifestyles.

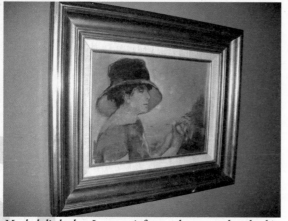

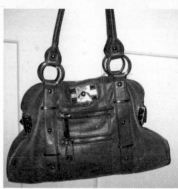

Love this purse because it is such a fun, unique color...

My dad died when I was an infant and my mom bought this painting because, as a young widow with a new baby, this painting touched her soul

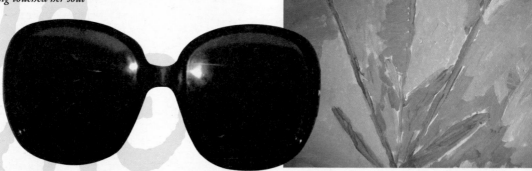

A "floral" painted by son Jack in the 3rd grade

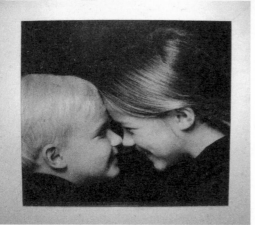

Photograph of my children, Jack and Caroline

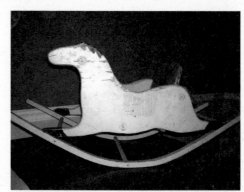

Antique rocking horse I bought in Canada... especially fun as it seats 2 toddlers

A FEW OF MY
Favorite Things

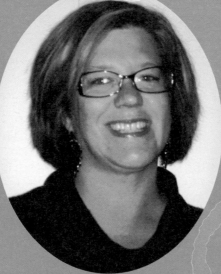

*Daughter Caroline's self-portrait
made in the 1st grade*

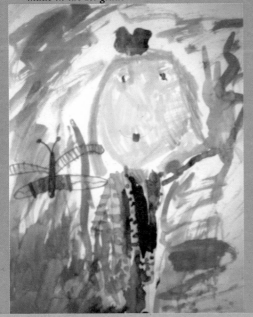

Katy Cross

Vice President, Regional Sales ~ Lifetime Television

*It's clear that among Katy's
favorites, the essence of childhood
is at the very core of her being.*

Childhood Obesity

If one of your favorite things is watching your children, grandchildren, nieces and nephews enjoy a healthy, active lifestyle... you can play an important part in this joy.

Teaching the young people in your life to enjoy fruits and vegetables, whole grains and low-fat dairy combined with a physically-active lifestyle can make you a hero and a favorite grown up.

Ask many children, tweens or teens about their favorite things, and the answers will likely involve an activity such as watching TV, playing video games or chatting on a computer. While there are benefits to each of these activities, they may be keeping children from healthy physical activities and may contribute to today's epidemic rates of childhood obesity.

Childhood obesity is usually caused by kids eating too much and exercising too little. Children can't change their exercise and eating habits by themselves. They need the help and support of their families and other caregivers. This is why successful prevention and treatment of childhood obesity starts at home.

Make it a Family Affair

Creating new family habits around healthy eating and increased physical activity can help a child lose weight and can also improve the health of other members of the family. Many communities are uniting to fight obesity among families, and particularly among children and adolescents.

Small Changes Can Bring Big Rewards

It's not a race. The first rule of change is to not make changes too quickly. It takes time and dedication to unlearn unhealthy behaviors and to develop new, healthy ones.

Think small. Small, gradual changes are easiest to follow and incorporate into your daily lives. And, small steps can result in big rewards over time. Pick a few small changes that seem doable, for example, turning off the TV during dinner, introducing a new fruit, vegetable or whole grain once a week or taking a walk after dinner.

> Set individual and family goals that are achievable and measurable.

Set individual and family goals that are achievable and measurable. Set specific goals for each family member, and then determine family goals. For example, your child's goal might be to eat fresh fruits and vegetables for afternoon snacks, and the family's goal might be to eat dinner outside of the home just once a week.

Childhood obesity crosses all socio-economic platforms. Unhealthy eating habits and lack of physical activity are becoming a problem for our entire society, which will lead to long-term medical and mental problems. The rates of diabetes, heart disease, certain cancers and arthritis all have increased and can be tracked back to overweight/obesity.

Changes must be made now to address the lack of education and access for healthy eating, and to encourage children and adults to make daily physical activity a priority in their lives.

The results from the newest study on childhood obesity indicate that the earlier kids begin to gain excess weight, the more likely they are to develop cardiovascular risk factors. You may be surprised to know that some of these risk factors can show up as early as age 7!

Because children grow at different rates, it isn't always easy to know when a child is obese or overweight. Ask your doctor to measure your child's BMI, or Body Mass Index, to determine if he or she is in a healthy range. Overcoming childhood obesity is something in which every adult can participate. Setting a good example of a healthy body image can be a strong, positive influence on young people. While obesity is an issue, we want to teach young people that a healthy body may not be what they see on TV in the form of anorexic images.

If a weight-loss program is necessary, involve the whole family in healthy habits so your child doesn't feel singled out. You can encourage healthy eating by serving more fruits and vegetables and buying fewer high-calorie, high-fat foods. Physical activity can also help your child overcome obesity or being overweight.

What Can You Do to Encourage Your Child?

- Encourage your children to take part in group activities with other children. Remember playing tag and kickball? Organize a neighborhood game and make it fun (and healthy) for all!

- Be sure to keep healthy snacks on hand and encourage your children to eat a minimum of 5 fruits and vegetable servings each day.

- Set a healthy example for your children. Make healthy eating and daily physical activity a priority for yourself and for your children. Most children need about 60 minutes of activity each day.

- Talk to your child's school to advocate for healthier school lunches and healthier snacks.

- Be sure your child eats breakfast every day. Skipping breakfast can leave your child hungry, tired and looking for less-healthy foods later in the day.

- Plan healthy meals and eat together as a family. Eating meals together helps children learn to enjoy a variety of foods.

- Eat fast food less often. When you visit a fast food restaurant, try the healthier options offered.

- Offer your child water or low-fat milk more often than fruit juice. Fruit juice is a healthy choice but is often high in calories.

- Try not to use food as a reward when encouraging kids to eat. Promising dessert to a child for eating vegetables, for example, sends the message that vegetables are less valuable than dessert. Kids learn to dislike foods they think are less valuable.

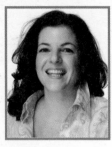

With practical tips, inspiring advice and real-life, actionable solutions, *Speaking of Women's Health* helps women across the nation become healthier on a daily basis. And because of that, FITNESS Magazine, whose mission is also to inspire women to make small, healthful changes and see big results, is honored to be a national sponsor of this unique organization. At FITNESS, we seek to change the way women think about almost every part of their lives, showing you that at every age working out and eating right can be a pleasure.

The book you hold in your hands makes those changes easy, providing a blueprint for exactly how to choose nutritious meals, reduce stress and manage your health. The best thing you can do with this book, aside from using it yourself, is to pass it along to a friend who has not yet seen that being healthy is not a goal, but an everyday habit that leads to success. Imagine a chain reaction, in which you offer just one recipe or piece of advice, that sparks another woman to change her daily habits. Now imagine that woman handing off that nugget of advice to a mom or sister. That chain reaction is what happens at *Speaking of Women's Health* events, where the message of healthy living resonates with real women and is then sent out into the farthest reaches of this country.

If you make the connection between living well and happiness, either through using the recipes specially created for this book by the FITNESS Healthy Test Kitchen for *Speaking of Women's Health*, or by integrating any of the other take-home messages here into your routines, our mission is complete.

I know you can do it, because I have seen readers who have lost weight, shaken off stress, found their inner athlete, changed their self-image and reinvented themselves, simply by starting with a few tiny changes. While watching a television program with my children, ages 11 and 9 recently, I heard a wonderful phrase: Imagine what you can do if you had no barriers, no limitations. Now, go out and do it.

Instead of waiting to live the life you've always wanted, stand up and take action now. Why wait? *Speaking of Women's Health* and FITNESS are here to help. We sincerely hope you enjoy the journey. I am lucky enough to have a job that allows me to pursue healthy goals, and teach them to my young children. I hope that you will make your own opportunity to do the same, and see how much happiness and success it brings in return.

All the best,

Denise Brodey
Editor-in-Chief
FITNESS Magazine

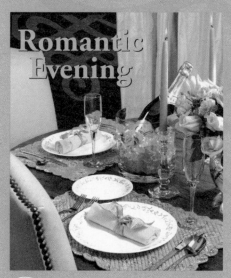

Romantic Evening

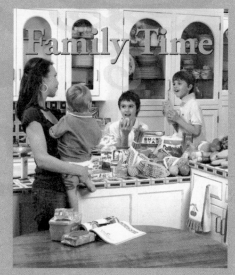

Family Time

A FEW OF OUR
Favorite Recipes

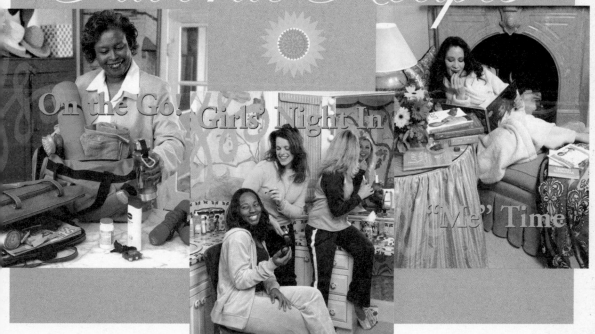

On the Go!

Girls' Night In

"Me" Time

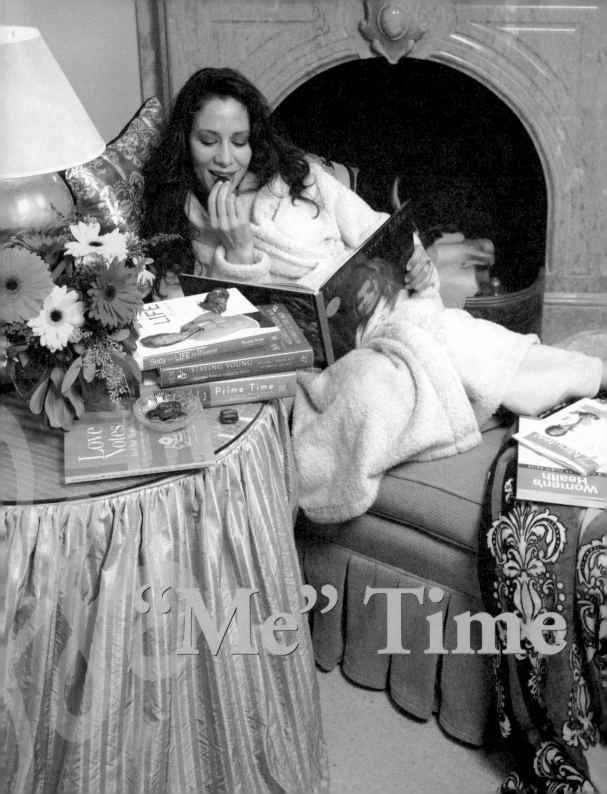

"Me" Time

A FEW OF OUR
Favorite Things

SPECIAL RECIPE SECTION - "ME" TIME

"Making time for myself is the most important thing I do. Sometimes my husband does the cooking, which is not all bad... as long as I make sure to set out the recipes!"

MINI-JOURNAL

Make a list of the recipes you might trust your husband with!

_____

_____

_____

_____

Ginger Chicken with Rice Noodles

Start to finish: 27 minutes
Makes: 4 servings

Nutrition facts per serving:
337 calories, 30 g protein,
34 g carbohydrate, 8 g fat
(1 g saturated), 3 g fiber.

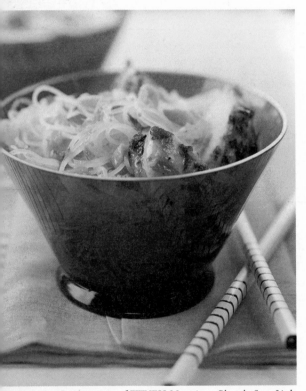

Recipe courtesy of FITNESS Magazine - Photo by Scott Little

INGREDIENTS

2	limes
4 Tbsp.	very finely chopped green onion
3 tsp.	grated fresh ginger
8	cloves garlic, minced
2 tsp.	olive oil
1/4 tsp.	salt
4	4 oz. skinless, boneless chicken breast halves
4 oz.	dried rice noodles
2 tsp.	packed brown sugar
1 cup	shredded carrots
4 Tbsp.	snipped fresh cilantro
4 Tbsp.	coarsely chopped peanuts

DIRECTIONS

In a small bowl combine green onion, ginger, 7 cloves of garlic, olive oil and salt. Rub ginger mixture evenly onto both sides of chicken. Place on the unheated rack of a broiler pan. Broil 4 to 5 inches from the heat for 12 to 15 minutes, turning once. Thinly slice chicken diagonally; keep warm. Meanwhile, cook noodles in a large saucepan in boiling water for 3 to 4 minutes or just until tender; drain. Finely shred two teaspoons lime peel. Squeeze 2 tablespoons juice from lime; set peel and juice aside. In a medium bowl stir together reserved lime peel and juice, brown sugar and the remaining 1 clove garlic until sugar is dissolved. Add hot cooked noodles, carrot, cilantro and peanuts; toss gently to coat. Spoon hot noodle mixture onto plates; arrange chicken slices on top. Serve immediately.

Guilt-Free Double Chocolate Brownies

INGREDIENTS

1/4 cup	butter
2/3 cup	granulated sugar
1/2 cup	cold water
1 tsp.	vanilla
1 cup	all-purpose flour
1/4 cup	unsweetened cocoa powder
1 tsp.	baking powder
1/4 cup	miniature semi-sweet chocolate pieces
2 tsp.	powdered sugar
	Nonstick cooking spray

Start to finish: 35 minutes
Makes: 16 brownies

Nutrition facts per brownie:
111 calories, 1 g protein,
18 g carbohydrate, 4 g fat
(3 g saturated), 1 g fiber.

DIRECTIONS

Preheat the oven to 350°F. Lightly coat the bottom of a 9x9x2-inch baking pan with nonstick cooking spray, being careful not to coat sides of pan. In a medium saucepan melt butter; remove from heat. Stir in granulated sugar, water and vanilla. Mix in flour, cocoa powder and baking powder until combined. Add chocolate pieces. Pour batter into pan. Bake for 15 to 18 minutes or until a wooden toothpick inserted near the center comes out clean. Cool in pan on a wire rack. Cut into bars; sprinkle with powdered sugar.

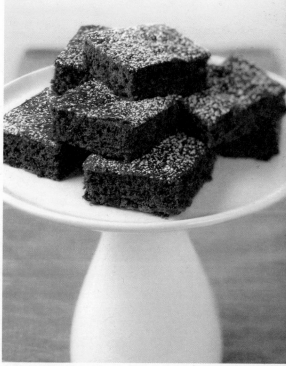

Recipe courtesy of FITNESS Magazine ~ Photo by Blaine Moats

Roasted Asparagus with Gruyere

Start to finish: 25 minutes
Makes: 6 servings

Nutrition facts per serving:
79 calories, 5 g protein,
6 g carbohydrate, 4 g fat
(1 g saturated), 2 g fiber.

INGREDIENTS

2 lbs.	fresh asparagus spears, trimmed
1	medium onion, cut into thin wedges
1	medium red or yellow sweet pepper, cut into thin strips
1 Tbsp.	olive oil
1/4 tsp.	salt
1/4 tsp.	ground black pepper
1 oz.	Gruyere or Swiss cheese, shredded (1/4 cup)

DIRECTIONS

Preheat the oven to 400°F. Place asparagus, onion, and sweet pepper in a 15x10x1-inch baking pan. Drizzle with olive oil; toss gently to coat. Spread in a single layer. Sprinkle with the salt and pepper. Roast, uncovered, about 20 minutes or until asparagus is crisp-tender, stirring once halfway through roasting time. Transfer to a serving platter; sprinkle with cheese. Let stand 2 minutes until cheese melts.

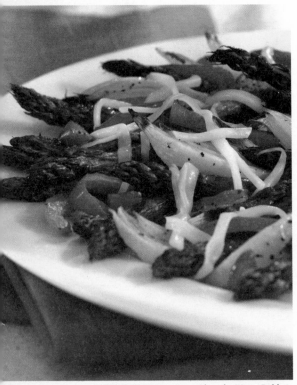

Recipe courtesy of FITNESS Magazine - Photo by Marty Baldwin

Strawberries with Lime Dipping Sauce

INGREDIENTS

1	8 oz. carton light dairy sour cream
2 Tbsp.	powdered sugar
2 tsp.	finely shredded lime peel
1 Tbsp.	lime juice
3 cups	strawberries

Prep: 10 minutes
Makes: 4 servings

Nutrition facts per serving:
128 calories, 3 g protein,
17 g carbohydrate, 6 g fat
(4 g saturated), 2 g fiber.

DIRECTIONS

For lime dipping sauce, in a small bowl stir together sour cream, powdered sugar, lime peel, and lime juice. Wash strawberries, but do not remove stems; drain. Serve the strawberries with the lime dipping sauce.

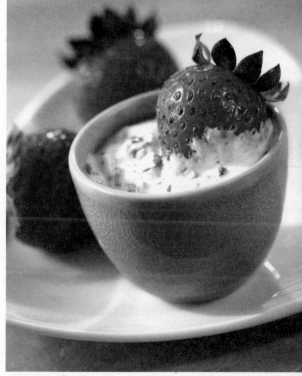

Recipe courtesy of FITNESS Magazine ~ Photo by Scott Little

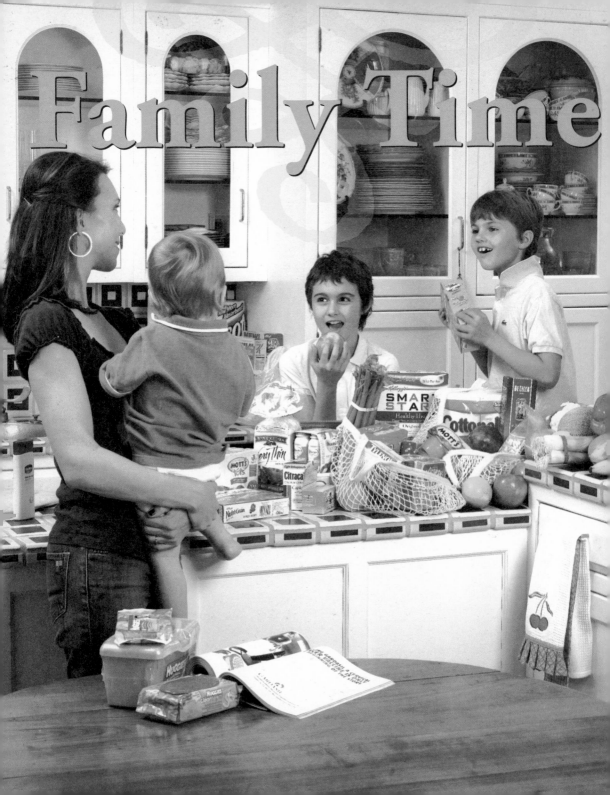

Family Time

A FEW OF OUR
Favorite Things

"One of my favorite things is to spend time with my family. Whether it's putting the groceries away, playing a board game or even making dinner, my time with my kids is golden."

MINI-JOURNAL
Make a list of the recipes your kids love that you already make.

_____

_____

_____

_____

Eggs and Canadian Bacon in Pita Pockets

Start to finish: 20 minutes
Makes: 4 servings

Nutrition facts per serving:
214 calories, 19 g protein,
19 g carbohydrate, 7 g fat
(3 g saturated), 2 g fiber.

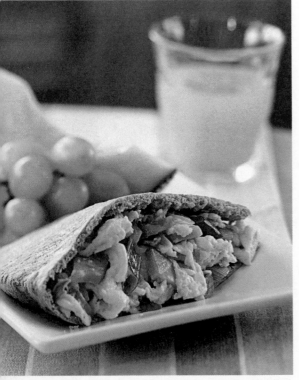

Recipe courtesy of FITNESS Magazine - Photo by Peter Krumhardt

INGREDIENTS

2	eggs
4	egg whites
4 oz.	Canadian-style bacon, finely chopped
2 Tbsp.	water
2 Tbsp.	snipped fresh chives
1/4 tsp.	salt
2	whole-wheat pitas
1/2 cup	shredded reduced-fat cheddar cheese
	Nonstick cooking spray

DIRECTIONS

In a small bowl beat together eggs, egg whites, Canadian bacon, water, chives and salt.

Lightly coat a nonstick skillet with egg mixture and cook until it begins to set on the bottom and around the edges. Using a spatula, lift and fold the partially cooked eggs so the uncooked portion flows underneath. Continue cooking about 2 minutes or until cooked through. Cut pitas in half crosswise and fill each with egg mixture. Sprinkle with cheese.

Chicken-Rice Soup

INGREDIENTS

2	14 oz. cans reduced-sodium chicken broth
1/2 tsp.	dried thyme or basil, crushed
4 cloves	garlic, minced
2	14 1/2 oz. cans petite diced tomatoes, undrained
1	9 oz. package frozen, chopped cooked chicken breast
1	8.8 oz. pouch cooked long grain & wild rice
1 cup	chopped zucchini
1/4 tsp.	ground black pepper
1 Tbsp.	Madeira or dry sherry (optional)

Start to finish: 20 minutes
Makes: 6 servings

Nutrition facts per serving:
162 calories, 15 g protein,
20 g carbohydrate, 3 g fat
(1 g saturated), 2 g fiber.

DIRECTIONS

In a 4-quart Dutch oven combine chicken broth, thyme, and garlic; bring to boiling. Stir in undrained tomatoes, chicken, rice, zucchini, and pepper. Return to boiling; reduce heat. Simmer, covered, for 5 minutes. If desired, stir in Madeira. Heat through.

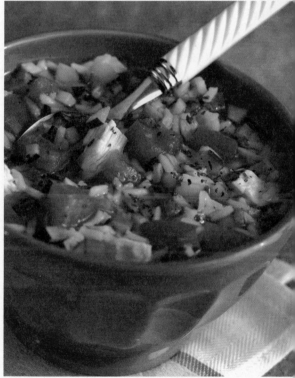

Recipe courtesy of FITNESS Magazine ~ Photo by Scott Little

Banana Oat Breakfast Cookies

Prep: 20 minutes
Bake: 14 minutes per batch
Makes: 12 servings

Nutrition facts per cookie:
230 calories, 6 g protein,
38 g carbohydrate, 6 g fat
(1 g saturated), 4 g fiber.

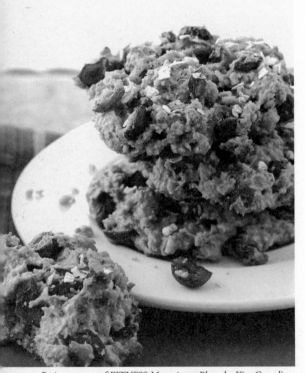

Recipe courtesy of FITNESS Magazine ~ Photo by Kim Cornelison

INGREDIENTS

	Nonstick cooking spray
1	large banana, mashed (1/2 cup)
1/2 cup	chunky natural peanut butter (unsalted and unsweetened) or regular chunky peanut butter
1/2 cup	honey
1 tsp.	vanilla
1 cup	regular rolled oats
1/2 cup	whole wheat flour
1/4 cup	non-fat dry milk powder
2 tsp.	ground cinnamon
1/4 tsp.	baking soda
1 cup	dried cranberries or raisins

DIRECTIONS

Preheat the oven to 350°F. Lightly coat two cookie sheets with cooking spray; set aside. In a large bowl stir together banana, peanut butter, honey, and vanilla. In a small bowl combine oats, flour, milk powder, cinnamon, and baking soda. Stir the oat mixture into the banana mixture until combined. Stir in dried cranberries.

Using a 1/4-cup measure, drop mounds of dough 3 inches apart on prepared baking sheets. With a thin metal or small plastic spatula dipped in water, flatten and spread each mound of dough to a 2 3/4-inch round, about 1/2-inch thick.

Bake, one sheet at a time, for **14 to 16** minutes or until browned. Transfer cookies to wire racks to cool completely. Store in an airtight container or resealable plastic bag for up to 3 days or freeze for up to 2 months; thaw before serving.

Taco Pizza

INGREDIENTS

	Nonstick cooking spray
1	1lb. loaf frozen whole wheat bread dough, thawed
1 cup	shredded reduced-fat cheddar cheese (4 ounces)
12 oz.	extra-lean ground beef
1	medium onion, chopped
2/3 cup	bottled chunky salsa
2	medium tomatoes, chopped
1 cup	shredded lettuce and/or spinach
1 cup	baked tortilla chips, coarsely crushed
	Light dairy sour cream and/or bottled chunky salsa (optional)

DIRECTIONS

Preheat the oven to 425°F. Lightly coat a 12-inch pizza pan with nonstick cooking spray. Pat dough evenly into prepared pan, extending edges over pan slightly. Sprinkle half of the cheese in a thin strip around the edge of the dough. Moisten edge of dough. Fold down edge over cheese and seal tightly to enclose the cheese. Prick crust all over with a fork. Bake for 10 minutes.

Meanwhile, in a large skillet cook the beef and onion until meat is brown and onion is tender. Drain off fat. Stir in 2/3 cup salsa. Top hot crust with meat mixture. Bake 5 minutes more. Sprinkle with tomatoes and remaining cheese. Bake 1 to 2 minutes more or until cheese melts. To serve, top with lettuce and tortilla chips. If desired, serve with sour cream and/or additional salsa.

Prep: 30 minutes
Bake: 16 minutes
Makes: 4 servings

Nutrition facts per serving:
583 calories, 43 g protein, 74 g carbohydrate, 15 g fat (5 g saturated), 7 g fiber.

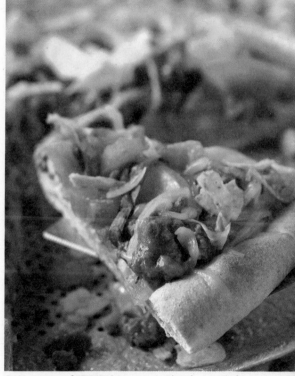

Recipe courtesy of FITNESS Magazine ~ Photo by Scott Little

Fruit-Filled Waffle Bowls

Start to finish: 10 minutes
Makes: 4 servings

Nutrition facts per serving:
141 calories, 5 g protein,
28 g carbohydrate, 1 g fat
(0 g saturated), 1 g fiber.

INGREDIENTS

1	4-serving-size package fat-free sugar-free reduced-calorie lemon or white chocolate instant pudding mix
2 cups	fat-free milk
4	waffle ice cream bowls or large waffle ice cream cones
1 cup	fresh fruit (such as blueberries, sliced kiwifruit, sliced strawberries, sliced bananas, or raspberries)
	Fresh mint leaves (optional)

DIRECTIONS

Prepare pudding according to package directions using the milk. Spoon fruit into waffle bowls or cones. Top with pudding. If desired, garnish with fresh mint leaves.

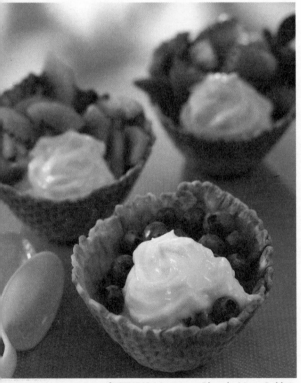

Recipe courtesy of FITNESS Magazine - Photo by Marty Baldwin

Saucy Chicken Parmesan

INGREDIENTS

4	small skinless, boneless chicken breast halves (about 1 pound)
	Nonstick cooking spray
1	slightly beaten egg white
3/4 cup	cornflakes, crushed (about 1/3 cup)
2 Tbsp.	grated Parmesan cheese
1/4 tsp.	dried Italian seasoning, basil, or oregano, crushed
1/8 tsp.	black pepper
1 1/3 cups	spaghetti sauce
4 oz.	whole-wheat spaghetti, fettuccine, or other pasta, cooked and drained

Start to finish: 35 minutes
Makes: 4 servings

Nutrition facts per serving:
355 calories, 34 g protein, 39 g carbohydrate, 7 g fat (1 g saturated), 4 g fiber.

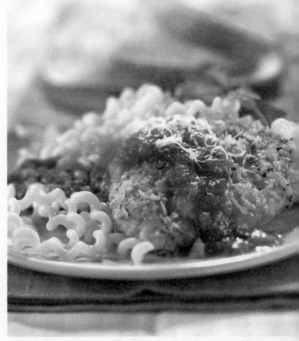

Recipe courtesy of FITNESS Magazine ~ Photo by Marty Baldwin

DIRECTIONS

Preheat the oven to 400°F. Place each chicken breast half between 2 pieces of plastic wrap; pound lightly with the flat side of a meat mallet (or rolling pin) to flatten to about 1/2 inch thick. Remove plastic wrap. Lightly coat a shallow baking pan with cooking spray; set aside. In a dish, combine egg white and one tablespoon water. In another dish combine crushed cornflakes, Parmesan cheese, Italian seasoning and pepper. Dip chicken pieces into egg, then coat with crumb mixture. Place chicken in pan and bake 15 minutes or until it's tender and no longer pink.

Meanwhile, in a small saucepan, warm spaghetti sauce over low heat. Divide pasta among 4 plates. Add chicken and spoon spaghetti sauce over it.

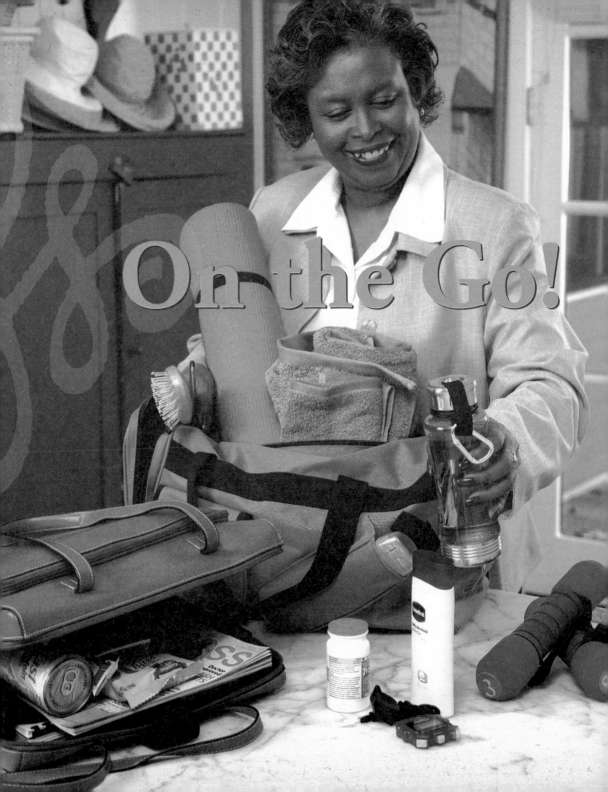

On the Go!

A FEW OF OUR
Favorite Things

SPECIAL RECIPE SECTION - ON THE GO

*"My favorite thing is to get
to the gym before I go to work.
That way, I'm feeling great, ready to go
and at the top of my game. Eating
smart is part of that for me."*

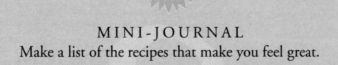

MINI-JOURNAL
Make a list of the recipes that make you feel great.

_____

_____

_____

_____

Cobb Salad Wraps

Start to finish: 20 minutes
Makes: 4 servings

Nutrition facts per serving:
357 calories, 29 g protein,
35 g carbohydrate, 11 g fat
(4 g saturated), 3 g fiber.

INGREDIENTS

1/2 cup	reduced-fat blue cheese or ranch salad dressing
4	8- to 10-inch whole wheat or tomato-flavored flour tortillas
4	romaine lettuce leaves, ribs removed
4	slices bacon, cooked
4	green onions cut into thin strips
2	Roma tomatoes, seeded and cut into thin wedges
1/2 cup	shredded reduced-fat mozzarella cheese
1 cup	cooked chicken breast, shredded

DIRECTIONS

Spread salad dressing over 1 side of each tortilla. Top with lettuce, bacon, green onions, tomato, cheese and shredded chicken. Roll tightly and serve.

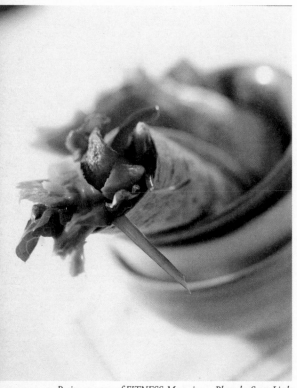

Recipe courtesy of FITNESS Magazine - Photo by Scott Little

Harvest Bran Muffins

INGREDIENTS

Nonstick cooking spray

1	14 oz. package oat bran muffin mix
1/3 cup	finely shredded carrot
1/4 cup	snipped dried apples
1/4 cup	dried cranberries or coarsely chopped dried tart cherries
3 Tbsp.	finely chopped walnuts

Start to finish: 30 minutes
Makes: 12 servings

Nutrition facts per serving:
161 calories, 3 g protein,
28 g carbohydrate, 4 g fat
(1 g saturated), 2 g fiber.

DIRECTIONS

Preheat oven to 400°F. Coat 12 two-and-a-half-inch muffin cups with nonstick cooking spray; set aside. Prepare muffin mix according to package directions; fold in carrot, dried apples, and cranberries. Divide evenly among prepared muffin cups and sprinkle with nuts.

Bake for 15 to 18 minutes or until golden. Cool in pan on wire rack for 5 minutes; remove from muffin cups and serve.

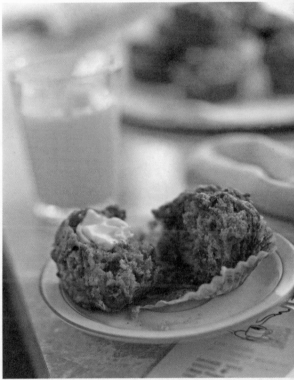

Recipe courtesy of FITNESS Magazine ~ Photo by Peter Krumhardt

Roast Beef Sandwiches with Horseradish Slaw

Start to finish: 15 minutes
Makes: 4 servings

Nutrition facts per serving:
255 calories, 17 g protein,
30 g carbohydrate, 6 g fat
(2 g saturated), 2 g fiber.

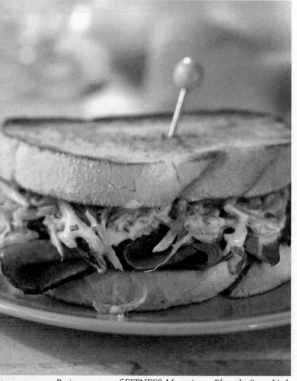

Recipe courtesy of FITNESS Magazine - Photo by Scott Little

INGREDIENTS

1/3 cup	light dairy sour cream
2 Tbsp.	snipped fresh chives
2 Tbsp.	spicy brown mustard
1 tsp.	prepared horseradish
1/2 tsp.	sugar
1/4 tsp.	salt
1 cup	packaged shredded broccoli (broccoli slaw mix)
8 oz.	thinly-sliced cooked roast beef
8	1/2-inch slices sourdough bread, toasted

DIRECTIONS

In a medium bowl combine sour cream, chives, mustard, horseradish, sugar and salt. Add shredded broccoli; toss to coat. Divide roast beef among four slices of bread. Top with broccoli mixture; finish with remaining bread slices.

Double Oat Granola

INGREDIENTS

	Nonstick cooking spray
2 1/2 cups	regular rolled oats
1 cup	toasted oat bran cereal
1/2 cup	toasted wheat germ
1/3 cup	pecans, coarsely chopped
1/2 cup	unsweetened applesauce
2 Tbsp.	honey
1 Tbsp.	canola oil
1/4 tsp.	ground cinnamon
1/3 cup	snipped dried cranberries, snipped dried tart cherries, and/or dried blueberries

Prep: 15 minutes
Bake: 40 minutes
Makes: 10 (1/2 cup) servings

Nutrition facts per serving:
257 calories, 9 g protein,
41 g carbohydrate, 8 g fat
(1 g saturated), 6 g fiber.

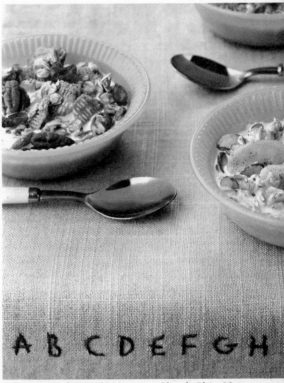

DIRECTIONS

Preheat the oven to 325°F. Lightly coat a 15x10x1-inch baking pan with nonstick cooking spray; set aside. In a large bowl stir together oats, oat bran cereal, wheat germ, and pecans. In a small bowl stir together applesauce, honey, oil, and cinnamon. Pour applesauce mixture over cereal mixture. Using a wooden spoon, stir until applesauce is evenly distributed.

Spread granola evenly onto prepared pan. Bake about 40 minutes or until golden brown, stirring every 10 minutes. Stir in dried fruit. Transfer to a large piece of foil; cool completely. Store in an airtight container for up to 2 weeks.

Recipe courtesy of FITNESS Magazine ~ Photo by Blaine Moats

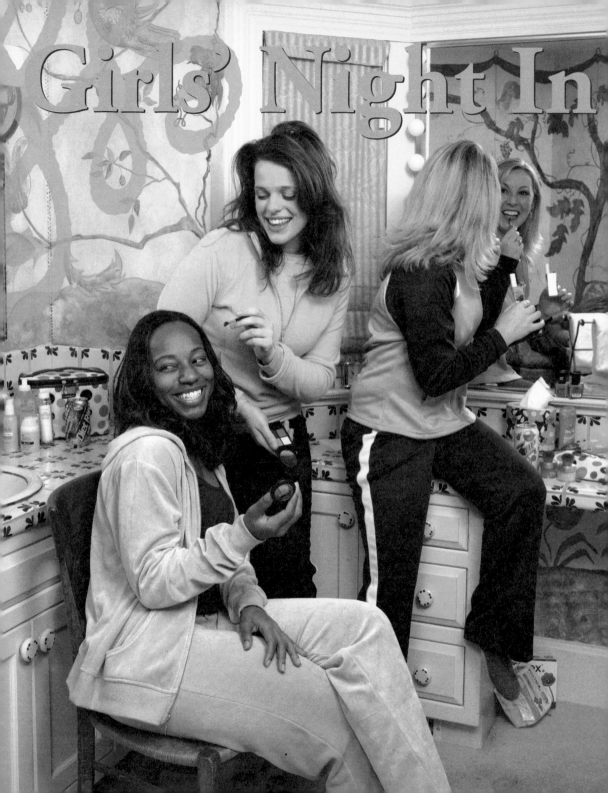

Girls' Night In

A FEW OF OUR
Favorite Things

"Getting together with my friends tops my list of favorites. Sometimes we cook up a storm, sometimes we just play. And sometimes, it's like we're 17 all over again!"

MINI-JOURNAL

Make a list of the recipes your girlfriends love to make.

_____

_____

_____

_____

Asian Spring Rolls

Start to finish: 30 minutes
Makes: 4 servings

Nutrition facts per serving:
207 calories, 15 g protein,
28 g carbohydrate, 3 g fat
(1 g saturated), 3 g fiber.

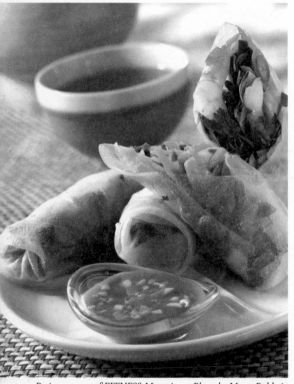

Recipe courtesy of FITNESS Magazine - Photo by Marty Baldwin

INGREDIENTS

8	8-inch round spring roll wrappers
2 cups	shredded Bibb lettuce (1 small head)
8 oz.	fresh or frozen cooked, peeled and de-veined shrimp, coarsely chopped
1 cup	shredded carrot
1/4 cup	sliced green onion
2 Tbsp.	chopped fresh cilantro
5 Tbsp.	bottled peanut sauce
2 Tbsp.	seasoned rice vinegar

DIRECTIONS

Fill a shallow dish with warm water. Dip each spring roll wrapper in water; place between damp paper towels for 10 minutes.

Meanwhile, in a large bowl combine lettuce, shrimp, carrot, green onion and cilantro. Add 2 tablespoons peanut sauce and 1 tablespoon rice vinegar. Toss to coat.

In a small bowl stir together the remaining 3 tablespoons peanut sauce and 1 tablespoon rice vinegar; set aside. Place about 1/2 cup of the shrimp mixture about 1/2 inch from bottom edge of one of the moistened spring roll wrappers. Fold bottom edge of the wrapper over the filling. Fold sides over and roll up. Repeat with remaining filling and wrappers. Cut them in half; serve with dipping sauce.

Oven-Fried Onion Rings

INGREDIENTS

	Nonstick cooking spray
3/4 cup	fine dry bread crumbs
3 Tbsp.	melted butter
1/4 tsp.	salt
2	medium sweet onions, cut into 1/4-inch slices and separated into rings
2	egg whites, slightly beaten

Prep: 25 minutes
Bake: 10 minutes
Makes: 6 servings

Nutrition facts per serving:
147 calories, 4 g protein,
18 g carbohydrate, 7 g fat
(4 g saturated), 1 g fiber.

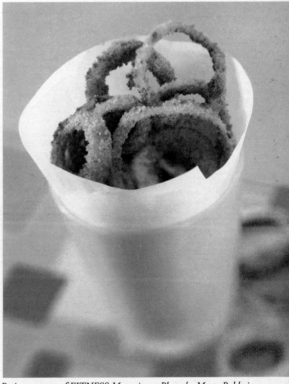

DIRECTIONS

Preheat the oven to 450°F. Lightly coat a very large baking sheet with cooking spray. In a small bowl stir together bread crumbs, melted butter, and salt. Spread about one-fourth of the crumb mixture on a sheet of waxed paper. Using a fork, dip the onion rings in the egg whites, then in the bread crumb mixture. Replace waxed paper and add more of the crumb mixture as needed.* Arrange the coated onion rings in a single layer on the prepared baking sheet. Bake for 10 to 12 minutes or until the coating is crisp and golden.

*Note: *The crumb mixture will not stick if combined with egg white mixture. Use one-fourth of the crumb mixture and a clean sheet of waxed paper at a time.*

Recipe courtesy of FITNESS Magazine ~ Photo by Marty Baldwin

Cheese and Bean Quesadillas

Start to finish: 30 minutes
Makes: 4 servings

Nutrition facts per serving:
217 calories, 11 g protein,
30 g carbohydrate, 6 g fat
(3 g saturated), 3 g fiber.

INGREDIENTS

1/4 cup	canned fat-free refried beans
4	8-inch whole wheat or regular flour tortillas
3/4 cup	shredded reduced-fat cheddar cheese (3 ounces)
1/4 cup	bottled chunky salsa

DIRECTIONS

Spread 1 tablespoon of the refried beans on one half of a tortilla. Place bean-topped tortilla, bean side up, in a medium skillet or on a griddle. Sprinkle one-quarter of the cheese over the bean-topped tortilla. Cook over medium heat about 3 minutes or until cheese begins to melt. Fold tortilla in half. Turn and cook 1 to 2 minutes more or until golden brown. Repeat with remaining refried beans, tortillas, and cheese. To serve, cut each quesadilla into thirds. Serve with salsa.

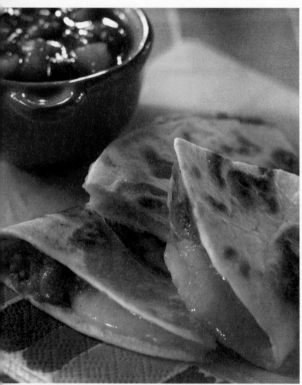

Recipe courtesy of FITNESS Magazine - Photo by Marty Baldwin

Star Fruit Salad

INGREDIENTS

1/4 cup	raspberry vinegar or red wine vinegar
3 Tbsp.	olive oil
1 Tbsp.	honey
1	10 oz. package torn mixed Italian blend salad greens
1	medium star fruit (carambola), thinly sliced
1/2	medium red onion, thinly sliced
	Fresh raspberries (optional)

DIRECTIONS

In a screw-top jar combine vinegar, oil, and honey. Cover and shake well. In a very large bowl toss salad greens with star fruit and onion. Shake dressing well and pour over salad mixture. Toss lightly to coat. If desired, garnish with fresh raspberries.

Start to finish: 15 minutes
Makes: 6 servings

Nutrition facts per serving:
89 calories, 1 g protein,
6 g carbohydrate, 7 g fat
(1 g saturated), 1 g fiber.

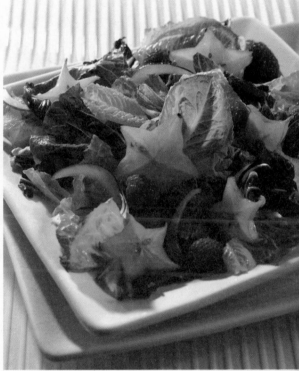

Recipe courtesy of FITNESS Magazine ~ Photo by Marty Baldwin

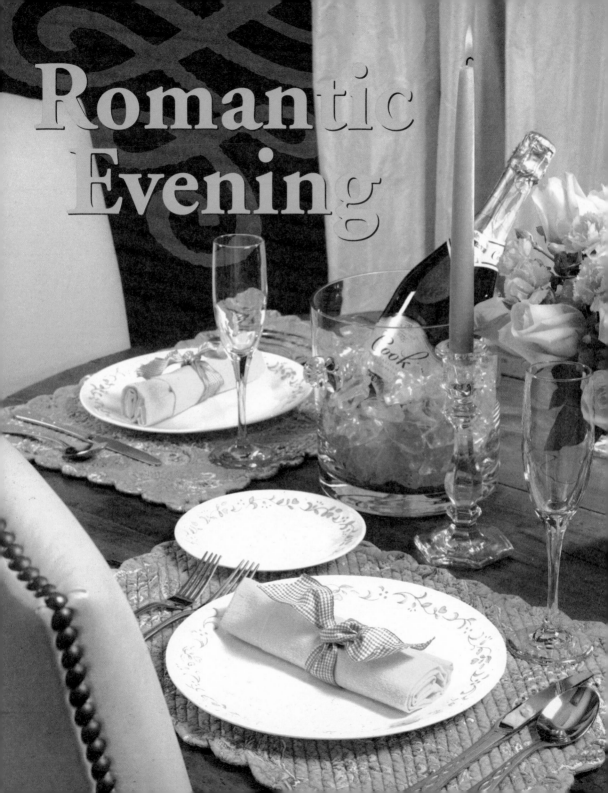

Romantic Evening

A FEW OF OUR
Favorite Things

"There's nothing I like more than a special night in. I make a really delicious dinner, light some candles and turn off the television! It works wonders."

MINI-JOURNAL

Make a list of the recipes you enjoy for your special nights.

_____

_____

_____

_____

Roast Tarragon Chicken

Start to finish: 55 minutes
Makes: 4 servings

Nutrition facts per serving:
382 calories, 39 g protein,
12 g carbohydrate, 19 g fat
(4 g saturated), 1 g fiber.

INGREDIENTS

3 Tbsp.	olive oil
2 1/2 tsp.	dried tarragon, rosemary, or thyme, crushed
2 cloves	minced garlic
1/2 tsp.	coarsely ground black pepper
1/4 tsp.	salt
1 lb.	cherry tomatoes
8	small shallots, trimmed
2 1/2 to 3 lbs.	chicken pieces (breasts, thighs, and drumsticks), skin removed

DIRECTIONS

Preheat the oven to 375°F. In a medium bowl, stir together oil, tarragon, garlic, pepper and salt. Add tomatoes and shallots; toss gently to coat. Use a slotted spoon to remove tomatoes and shallots from bowl, reserving oil mixture. Place chicken in a shallow roasting pan, brush chicken with reserved oil mixture and roast for 20 minutes. Add the shallots; roast for 15 minutes. Add the tomatoes; roast for 10 to 12 minutes or until chicken and vegetables are tender.

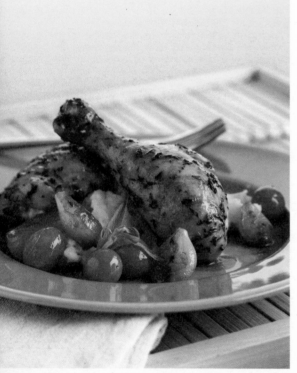

Recipe courtesy of FITNESS Magazine - Photo by Robert Jacobs

Salmon with Feta and Pasta

INGREDIENTS

12 oz.	fresh or frozen skinless salmon fillet
1/4 tsp.	salt
8 oz.	dried whole wheat or regular rotini pasta
	Nonstick cooking spray
2 cloves	garlic, minced
4	plum tomatoes, chopped
1 cup	sliced green onions
1/3 cup	sliced pitted ripe olives
3 Tbsp.	snipped fresh basil
1/2 tsp.	coarsely ground black pepper
2 tsp.	olive oil
1	4 oz. package crumbled reduced-fat feta cheese
	Fresh basil sprigs (optional)

Start to finish: 25 minutes
Makes: 4 servings

Nutrition facts per serving:
460 calories, 31 g protein,
51 g carbohydrate, 18 g fat
(5 g saturated), 9 g fiber.

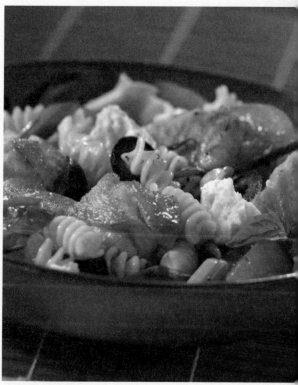

Recipe courtesy of FITNESS Magazine - Photo by Mike Dieter

DIRECTIONS

Thaw fish, if frozen. Rinse fish; pat dry. Cut into 1-inch pieces. Sprinkle fish with salt. Cook pasta according to pasta directions. Drain. Keep warm.

Meanwhile, lightly coat a large nonstick skillet with cooking spray. Heat skillet over medium-high heat. Add garlic. Cook and stir for 15 seconds. Add fish to skillet. Cook fish for 4 to 6 minutes or until fish flakes easily when tested with a fork, turning fish pieces occasionally. Stir in tomatoes, onions, olives, snipped basil, and pepper. Heat through. In a large bowl toss together hot pasta, olive oil, salmon mixture, and cheese. If desired, garnish with basil sprigs.

Lemon-Marinated Baby Vegetables

Prep: 20 minutes
Chill: 2 hours
Makes: 8 servings

Nutrition facts per serving:
57 calories, 2 g protein,
9 g carbohydrate, 2 g fat
(0 g saturated), 3 g fiber.

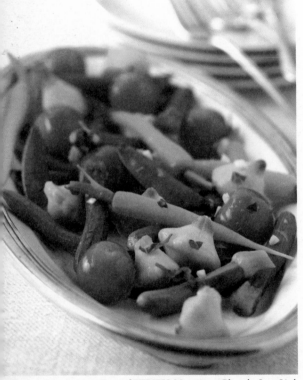

Recipe courtesy of FITNESS Magazine ~ Photo by Scott Little

INGREDIENTS

2 lbs.	baby whole fresh vegetables (such as carrots, zucchini, and/or yellow summer squash)
8 oz.	fresh sugar snap peas
12	cherry tomatoes
1/2 tsp.	finely shredded lemon peel
2 Tbsp.	lemon juice
2 Tbsp.	water
1 Tbsp.	olive oil
1 Tbsp.	snipped fresh basil or oregano
1 tsp.	Dijon-style mustard
1 clove	garlic, minced
1/2 tsp.	salt

DIRECTIONS

In a covered large saucepan cook vegetables in a small amount of lightly salted boiling water for 3 minutes. Add peas. Cook, covered, about 2 minutes more or until vegetables are crisp-tender; drain. Rinse with cold water; drain again. Transfer to a large bowl. Add cherry tomatoes.

Meanwhile, for dressing, in a screw-top jar combine lemon peel, lemon juice, the water, oil, basil, mustard, garlic, and salt. Cover and shake well to combine. Pour dressing over vegetables; toss gently to coat. Cover and chill for 2 to 24 hours.

INGREDIENTS

1/2	of a 3-ounce package ladyfingers, cubed (12 halves)
1/4 cup	brewed espresso or strong coffee
1/4	of an 8 oz. package reduced-fat cream cheese (Neufchatel), softened
1/2 cup	light dairy sour cream
3 Tbsp.	sugar
1 tsp.	vanilla
1/2 tsp.	unsweetened cocoa powder

Prep: 20 minutes
Chill: 1 hour
Makes: 4 servings

Nutrition facts per serving:
149 calories, 3 g protein,
18 g carbohydrate, 7 g fat
(4 g saturated), 0 g fiber.

DIRECTIONS

Divide ladyfinger cubes among four 4- to 6-ounce dessert dishes. Drizzle ladyfinger cubes with espresso. Set aside. In a medium bowl beat together cream cheese, sour cream, sugar, and vanilla. Beat until smooth. Spoon cream cheese mixture over ladyfinger cubes. Cover and chill for 1 to 24 hours. Just before serving, sprinkle with cocoa powder.

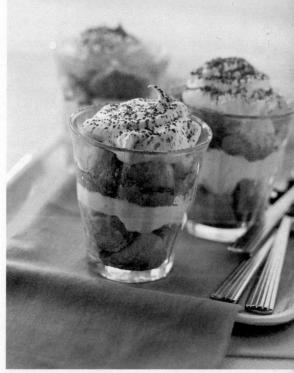

Recipe courtesy of FITNESS Magazine ~ Photo by Peter Krumhardt

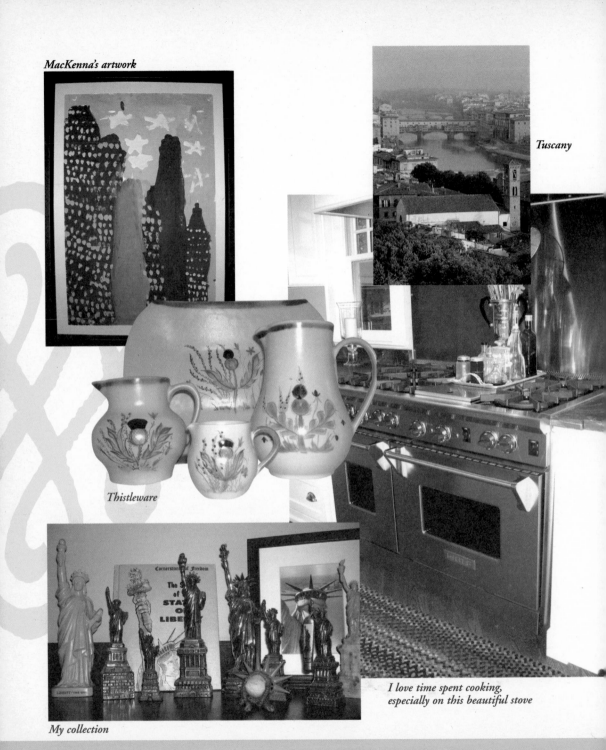

MacKenna's artwork

Tuscany

Thistleware

My collection

I love time spent cooking,
especially on this beautiful stove

92

Favorite Things

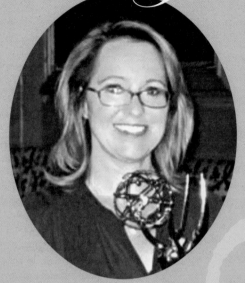

Margaret Asselin-Woods

Marketing Director, Dove Chocolates ~ MasterFood

*When Margaret sent us her favorite things,
there were several pictures of her Statue of Liberty collection.
We were particularly taken by a comment she wrote,
"My Statue of Liberty collection is my favorite art.
It means freedom to be me and a woman of strength."
Margaret Asselin-Woods certainly represents our motto,
"Be Strong. Be Healthy. Be in Charge."*

De-Mess to De-Stress

Many women tell us that one of their favorite things is a space of peace and quiet, free from the stresses of every day. For many of us, we think of home as a refuge, safe from the demands of life.

If your home is cluttered, somewhat disorganized or overstuffed, relaxation can be virtually impossible. Living in a cluttered home can create constant low-grade stress and subtly, but steadily, drain your energy.

As your life gets fuller, keeping order should become a priority. **The good news is...** a few simple strategies can put you on the path toward managing your constantly-evolving life.

Keep your body in great shape year-round.

Maintain a healthy lifestyle and diet (see Chapter 5). Get regular health screenings. Be sure to be physically active and strive to stay focused on the positives in your life including family and loved ones, a circle of supportive friends, hobbies and leisure activities that bring you joy.

Small Steps = Big Rewards

- Many experts tell us that the way we start our day can have an impact on the rest of the day. Begin with taking just a moment after the alarm goes off and before you get out of bed. Stretch. Breathe. Raise your arms one at a time and reach for the sun. Alternate between stretching and flexing your outstretched legs and feet. Keep breathing. Just 5 minutes will help prepare your body (and soul) for the day. Next... the shower. The warm water will help relax your muscles and help to release stored tension and enable you to start the day feeling more relaxed, at peace, and ready to handle what comes your way.

- **Don't forget to refuel.** Breakfast is "the most important meal of the day" for a very good reason: a healthy meal in the morning can balance your blood sugar levels and give you the sustenance you need to handle physical and mental activities. Without it, you will be less resilient, both physically and mentally. Be sure to include fiber, protein and fruit.

- **Take a walk.** Consider walking the kids to the bus stop or parking a few blocks from work. Even if it's as simple as taking the stairs instead of the elevator at work... get moving! Aerobic activities such as walking cause your heart to pump faster, infusing extra oxygen into your blood and throughout your body.

deMess = deStress

Organization is not a one-time deal... it requires a full-fledged strategy to bring control and calm to your household and your time. Begin with these simple ideas:

- First... Survey your belongings: Examine what you have and how you store it. Sell or donate what you don't use.

- Keep things you use frequently in easily-accessible places.

- Get boxes for items you use only seasonally or will be storing, such as holiday decorations or sports gear. Set up a box for items that need repair.

- Keep important papers (birth and marriage certificates, citizenship papers, real estate deeds) in a fireproof safe box. Create a file for personal documents such as insurance policies, credit reports, Social Security cards and the like.

- Develop a finance file for unpaid bills, bank statements and income tax papers.

- Store home-maintenance papers (warranties, receipts, manuals) in another place.

- Create consistent, regular "systems" for who will do what and when. Divide household chores, and schedule when they should be accomplished.

- Assign certain days for paying bills. Many women tell us that online or computer-bill paying is a terrific time saver.

- Manage your time efficiently by planning activities on a calendar and making to-do lists. Take advantage of days off or weekends to plan meals for the week ahead, and complete your grocery list at the same time. Keep track of all family activities and rehearsals, practices and work schedules on one master sheet.

Now that you've got the basics in place, use them wisely. Use this simple plan... touch things only once. That means, when you get the mail each day, immediately eliminate what is waste and put each correspondence in its place (remember to shred and recycle papers). The key is to do it now... don't start a pile that you'll "deal with" later. That leads to clutter!

Put things you use back in their place right away. Get into the habit of immediately cleaning up after yourself.

Take a few minutes at the end of each day to plan for the next day. Consider making lunches while dinner is in the oven. Ask the kids to help by making sandwiches, organizing the lunch boxes or gathering snacks. Think through clothing options for yourself and others. Consider keeping a box by the door where children leave their gym bags, homework or book bags ready to go before the morning rush.

Overloaded by e-mail?

Take the same approach as outlined for regular mail... touch or read it only once. When you open an e-mail, assign it to a home, either a "needs attention" or an "action completed" folder. Make an effort to manage e-mails at specific times each day, rather than throughout the day.

As you develop stress-relieving practices in your daily life, you should experience less stress and be better able to handle the stress you do experience, leading to a happier, healthier life.

This is how I escape (bike) when I need a break

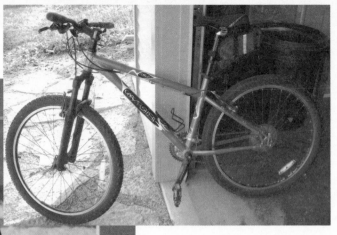

Picture of my son on the north shore of Oahu

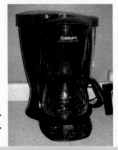

My dog, Scooby. She is always there to greet me, regardless of my day.

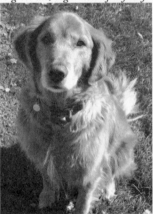

My favorite book

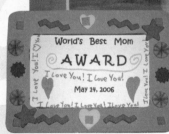

World's Best Mom – My son gave it to me for Mother's Day 2006

My 10 year-old coffee pot. So reliable, I can always count on it.

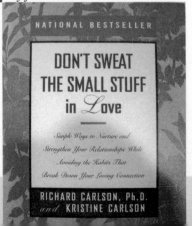

A FEW OF MY
Favorite Things

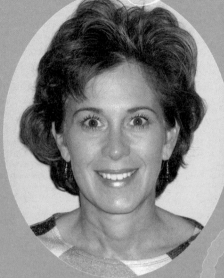

Kim Underhill

President, North American Family Care ~ Kimberly-Clark

*The day of my graduation,
I told myself... "Freeze this day in your
mind. Many good things are ahead."*

*As you can see from Kim's pictures of
her favorite things, she was right!*

Healthy Pregnancy

Girls in white dresses with blue satin sashes
Snowflakes that stay on my nose and eyelashes
Silver white winters that melt into springs

These are a few of my favorite things... and, of course, each is made better by the presence of children. Whether you're pregnant for the first time, or if you've been through this before... you'll want to give your baby a healthy start. Here are some tips to help ensure your own health, as well as that of your baby, for the next 9 months and beyond.

Off to a Healthy Start

Be sure to get prenatal care as soon as you think you're pregnant. It's important to both you and your baby. Most health care professionals recommend that women who are considering pregnancy, or are pregnant, begin taking a specially-formulated prenatal vitamin daily to ensure adequate (increased) intake of needed vitamins and minerals including folic acid, calcium, Vitamin D and iron.

If nausea and morning sickness are a problem, consider eating 5 or 6 small meals a day instead of 3 large ones. Pregnancy is not a time for dieting! Don't stop eating or start skipping meals as your weight increases. Both you and your baby need the calories and nutrition you receive from a healthy diet.

Drink extra fluids (water is best) throughout pregnancy to help your body keep up with the increases in your blood volume. Drink at least 6 to 8 glasses of water, fruit juice, or low-fat milk each day. A good way to know you're drinking enough fluid is when your urine looks almost clear or is very light yellow.

Help Ensure a Healthy Baby

Many prenatal vitamins contain 1 mg of folic acid. This is included in prenatal vitamins taken just before pregnancy and during the first few months of pregnancy to reduce the risk of birth defects of the brain and spine. Of course, always talk with your physician. It is also important to eat a healthy diet with fortified foods (enriched whole wheat and whole-grain products including cereals, rice, breads and pastas) and foods with natural sources of folate (orange juice, green leafy vegetables, beans, broccoli, asparagus, peas and lentils).

Nutrition During Pregnancy

Good nutrition is vitally important to both you and your baby. Your meals should include the 5 basic food groups. Each day you should get the following:

- 6-11 servings of grain products
- 3-5 servings of vegetables
- 2-4 servings of fruits
- 4-6 servings of milk and milk products
- 3-4 servings of meat and protein foods

Physical activity during pregnancy can benefit both you and your baby by lessening discomfort and fatigue, providing a sense of well-being, and increasing the likelihood of a quicker recovery after delivery. Light to moderate exercise during pregnancy strengthens the abdominal and back muscles, which helps to improve your posture. Practicing Yoga, walking, swimming and cycling on a stationary bicycle are usually safe exercises for pregnant women. But, always check with your doctor before beginning any kind of exercise, especially during pregnancy.

Finally... get your ZZZZZZZZs. Be sure to get plenty of rest. When resting, lie on your left side as often as possible, as it provides the best circulation to your baby and helps reduce swelling.

Let your physician know if you experience any of the following: Pain of any kind, strong cramps, uterine contractions at 20-minute intervals, vaginal bleeding, leaking of amniotic fluid, dizziness, fainting, shortness of breath, palpitations, tachycardia (rapid beating of the heart), constant nausea and vomiting, trouble walking, edema (swelling of joints), or if your baby has decreased activity.

Know Your Limits

- There is no safe amount of alcohol a woman can drink while pregnant.
- A recent study shows that caffeine, found in tea, coffee and soft drinks, significantly increased the occurrence of miscarriage. You may want to discuss the use of caffeine with your physician.
- Your pharmacist can be a helpful consultant regarding medications, over-the-counter cold and cough remedies, as well as herbs and vitamins.

A New Addition

Now is the perfect time to prepare yourself mentally for the change your life is about to experience. Spend quality time with "Dad." Educate yourself about pregnancy, birth, infancy and beyond. While nothing can prepare you for all of the joy you are about to experience, the more you know, the better prepared you will feel. Talk to your family about the kind of parent you hope to become.

If you already have children in the home, take extra care that they understand how a new baby may change things. Help young siblings to feel they are part of the baby's life from the beginning. Encourage them to ask questions and to play a role in your pregnancy. Discuss together how routines may change once the new baby comes home. This can go a long way toward solidifying your family as you are about to bring a new member into the fold.

R_x for Health

If you are taking prescription drugs, talk to your pharmacist or health care provider to make sure that none of these drugs will have a negative effect on your pregnancy. You can also ask about over-the-counter products and natural/herbal remedies. Read drug labels carefully. Avoid anything that is not recommended for pregnant women.

NOTE:
Please consult your doctor on any and all issues regarding your pregnancy. Although these may be good general pregnancy tips, every pregnancy is different, and each deserves the attention of a doctor or health care provider. Go to www.speakingofwomenshealth.com **for lots of great information on the growth of your baby over the 40 weeks of pregnancy, how your body changes, how to engage "Dad," and how to help prepare siblings.**

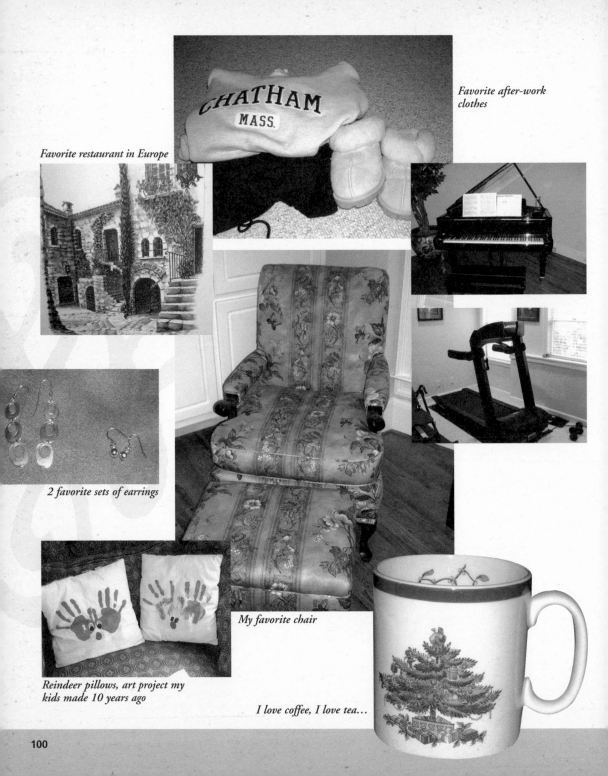

Favorite after-work clothes

Favorite restaurant in Europe

2 favorite sets of earrings

My favorite chair

Reindeer pillows, art project my kids made 10 years ago

I love coffee, I love tea...

A FEW OF MY
Favorite Things

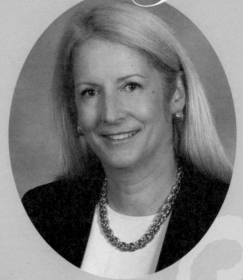

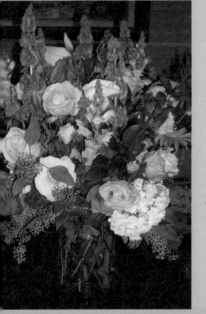

Fresh flowers in my office

Joanne Bauer

President ~ Kimberly-Clark Health Care

At Speaking of Women's Health, we're all about good health and we believe that an essential ingredient of good health is taking the time to relax and pamper yourself. From fresh flowers in her office, to her comfy clothes and cozy chair, Joanne really knows how to balance her life.

Healthy Baby Care

*Who can resist the smile of a baby or young child?
No matter what your age, hearing the laughter of a child or
seeing absolute joy in a sparkling eye and a toothless grin
is one of life's essential pleasures!*

If spending time with children is among your favorite things, this chapter will help you better understand how you can contribute to a child's well-being — whether you're a parent, grandparent, aunt, friend or neighbor… *"it takes a village to raise a child."*

Infancy

It's normal for new parents and caregivers to feel a mixture of excitement, joy and love along with some anxiety, fear and a little trepidation. However, with some technical and developmental know-how, coupled with the love and support of family, friends, time and patience, new parents will embrace this time. It's essential that new parents provide for baby's needs without sacrificing their own health and well-being. Now, more than ever, it is important that you maintain a healthy diet, get some exercise and set aside time for yourself. Learn to say "yes" to offers of respite, even if just long enough for a walk around the block or to pamper yourself with an uninterrupted bath or nap.

What to Feed

For about the first 5 or 6 months of life, babies get all of their nutrients from the milk they drink. The American Academy of Pediatrics strongly suggests breast feeding your newborn as the best option. Breast feeding has proven to provide your baby with the best nutrients and immunities. New parents have a few options about how to feed their infants. They can choose to breast feed, to pump breast milk (a nice option when others help care for baby) or to bottle-feed using specialized baby formula. Infants do not need any other food or water outside these 3 sources. For the first 3 months, parents and caregivers should follow the baby's signals about when they're hungry or full.

While each child is different, most babies can begin transitioning to solid foods at around 6 months. Caregivers may notice their infant watching adults eat and wanting to be involved at dining situations. In addition, babies may begin waking up in the middle of the night hungry again, even though they had been sleeping through the night for weeks or months. Discuss solid food introduction and options with your pediatrician to make sure that baby's unique nutritional and medical needs are being addressed.

One of baby's first solid foods is baby rice cereal mixed with formula or breast milk. Babies can now have breast milk or formula with cereal for 2 meals a day. After a few weeks or a month of feeding cereal, in addition to breast or bottles, you can begin gradually adding new foods. Doctors recommend trying only one new food a week to watch for any potential food allergies.

Just as nutrition is vital to infants' growth and development, sleep is also a main building block of life. When babies are born, their sleep patterns are not set and they need to be taught how to fall asleep. To help babies learn to soothe themselves to sleep, create a bedtime routine that will help relax them and transition them from day to night. This routine can include a warm bath, cuddling or soft music. It's never too early to begin reading to your baby. Teach babies to soothe themselves to sleep by putting them in their bed when they're full and drowsy but not yet asleep.

Send the message that nighttime is for sleeping, not for fun and play!

When infants cry in the middle of the night for a bottle or a diaper change, provide for those needs quickly and quietly. Babies should always be put down to sleep on their backs; never on their stomachs or on their sides.

Good nutrition, sleep, hygiene and basic medical care are essential for babies' overall health. Babies need to be loved and nurtured from birth to create a trusting bond between them and the adults who care for them. This will help babies create trust and interest in the world at large, enabling them to grow and to learn.

You can actually make diapering time fun!

The most valuable loving and teaching moments often come during everyday activities. Parents and caregivers should constantly talk to and interact with the baby. They can describe what they're doing while they do it and describe things in the environment. They can ask the baby questions, even if the baby can't yet respond. Caregivers can also sing, laugh, read and pray with the baby. Not only will this interaction improve social skills, it will also help develop the baby's language comprehension and expression skills.

Loving, nurturing, family playtime is fun for everyone. Parents and caregivers will enjoy the time that is dedicated to stimulating the baby's mind and senses. This is a perfect opportunity for the entire family to grow together and will set a precedent that can build and strengthen relationships that span into childhood and beyond.

Be sure to follow your pediatrician's or health care professional's advice regarding regularly-scheduled visits, vaccinations and growth and development checks.

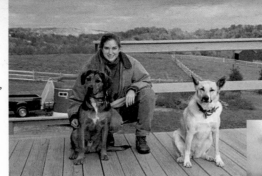

My pets are "rescues"

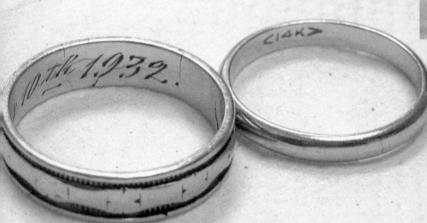

My grandmother's and mother's wedding rings

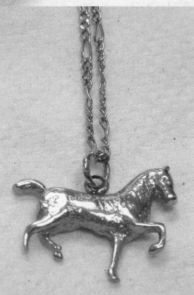

Horse pendant, a gift from my mother when I was 6

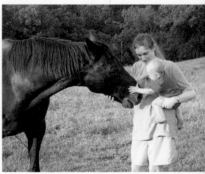

Sharing my love of horses

A FEW OF MY
Favorite Things

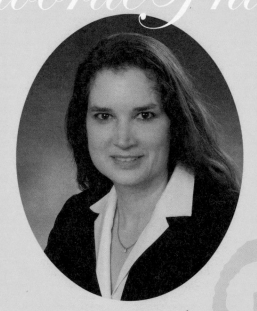

Karen Lindquist

Marketing Manager, HPV Franchise ~ Merck

"On the morning of my 6th birthday, my mother woke me with presents — a riding helmet and paddock boots. She drove me to a stable, where I took my first riding lesson. After the lesson, we stopped at a small jewelry store, where she bought me the pendant to remind me of this day. It was the beginning of my lifelong relationship with horses, leading me to become a veterinarian and to have the 4 horses I currently own."

Speaking to Girls About Health™

If you're a parent of a tween or teen, some time spent together may be among your favorite things to do.

There is great joy in watching them develop and mature into young adults. Along with this joy, there are bound to be confusing times. Self-esteem can be an issue at any age... luckily, problems are usually temporary! For "tweens" (ages 9–12) and teens who are still figuring out who they are and where they fit into the world, self-esteem is an important step to self-awareness. How a teen feels about herself can be related to many different factors — environment, body image, self-expectations, personal experiences, as well as parental expectations. Here are some steps for building positive self-esteem.

10 Tips for Growing Together, Connecting for Life™

Consider saying to your tweens and teens:

1. **Focus on your best attributes.** The outer you is changing every day, but by focusing on your talents, your skills, your character and your heart, you'll like yourself no matter how bad a hair day or acne issue you're having.

2. **Exercise!** You'll not only improve your body, but you'll relieve stress at the same time.

3. **Replace negative thoughts with positive ones.** Instead of criticizing yourself, give yourself a pat on the back.

4. **Be forgiving.** If your friends make mistakes, forgive them. Do the same for yourself.

5. **Speak up for yourself.** Don't be afraid to share your opinions and ideas. And, if someone tries to put you down, stand up to them.

6. **Every day, make a list** of 3 things about yourself that makes you happy.

7. **Don't be a perfectionist.** Remember, it's those little imperfections that make us unique and wonderful!

8. **Consider helping others,** like raising money for a cause you believe in. Once you start thinking about other people, you won't be so focused on your own problems.

9. **Surround yourself with friends** who love you for who you are, not what you wear or how you look.

10. **Have fun now!**

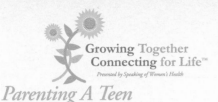

Growing Together Connecting for Life™

Presented by Speaking of Women's Health

Parenting A Teen

Help your teen develop and maintain a positive self-image. It starts with listening. Helping to guide them as they learn to make decisions and to have opinions of their own will enhance your image in their eyes. Spend time with your teen and let them feel that they are contributing to the family dynamic in a positive way.

What a parent can do to help a child develop a positive self-image:

- Teach children to change their "demands" to "preferences." Encourage them to work against frustration by setting a good example and reward them when they express their needs and desires appropriately.

- Encourage your children to ask for what they want assertively, pointing out that there is no guarantee that they will get it.

- Encourage your children to develop hobbies and interests that give them pleasure and that they can pursue independently.

- Let children settle their own disputes between siblings and friends alike.

- Help children learn to focus on their strengths by pointing out to them all the things they CAN do.

- Encourage your children to value themselves the way they'd like their friends to value them.

- Help your children think in terms of alternative options and possibilities rather than depending upon one option for satisfaction.

- Finally, enjoy your teen. It's far too easy to get caught up in the negative and forget to just enjoy the time you spend together.

So, what's the payoff?

Studies prove that teens with high self-esteem do better in school and enjoy it more and find it easier to make friends. They tend to have better relationships with peers and adults, feel happier, find it easier to deal with mistakes, disappointments and failures, and are more likely to stick with something until they succeed. Improving self-esteem takes work, but the payoff is feeling good about oneself and one's accomplishments.

Set a healthy example for your tweens and teens.

- Make positive statements about yourself in front of your child, rather than complaining about your weight, hair, job, etc.

- Exercise and enjoy physical activity.

- Eat a healthy, balanced nutritious diet. If you need to lose weight, do so in a healthy manner, rather than through fad or yo-yo dieting.

- Talk to your child about relationships and make an effort to be open-minded about her choice of friends.

- Help your teen set realistic expectations and establish time management skills.

- Set appropriate boundaries and communicate the importance of self-discipline.

- Ensure that your tween or teen takes responsibility for her actions, both good and bad.

- Listen, listen and listen to your children.

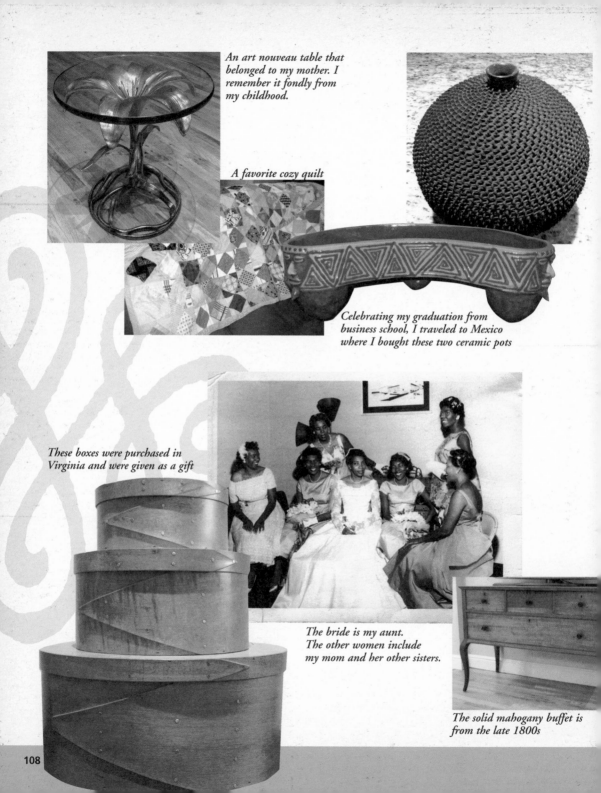

An art nouveau table that belonged to my mother. I remember it fondly from my childhood.

A favorite cozy quilt

Celebrating my graduation from business school, I traveled to Mexico where I bought these two ceramic pots

These boxes were purchased in Virginia and were given as a gift

The bride is my aunt. The other women include my mom and her other sisters.

The solid mahogany buffet is from the late 1800s

A FEW OF MY
Favorite Things

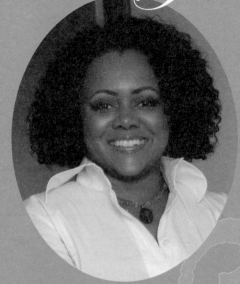

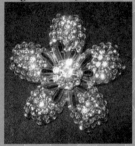

This beautiful vintage brooch from the designer/author June Ambrose

Kathryn Peeler

Senior Vice President, Global Marketing ~ SoftSheen-Carson

My mother's 18-carat gold bracelet was made in West Africa. She loved it very much, therefore my sisters also love it. We could not decide which of us should keep it... so each year, on Thanksgiving, we pass it on to the next sister so we all get to enjoy it.

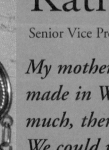

Prevent Cervical Cancer

If one of your favorite things is maintaining a healthy dialogue with your daughter and other young women in your life, this chapter may be a great resource.

An open and honest dialogue will help you become a woman of influence and a "favorite" for someone else.

Cervical cancer is caused by a group of viruses called the human papillomavirus (HPV). It has been estimated that up to 80% of all sexually-active women will be exposed to HPV during their lives. Surprisingly, about 1 in 4 American women under the age of 60 are infected with HPV. However, not all of these women will develop cervical cancer.

Fortunately, only 2 especially aggressive strains account for the majority of cervical cancer cases. In recent years, researchers have directed efforts to prevent HPV from causing cervical cancer.

Since the Pap test was introduced as a routine screening to detect abnormal, pre-cancerous and cancerous cells in the cervix, there has been a dramatic drop in the number of women who lose their lives to cervical cancer.

Only some women with pre-cancerous changes of the cervix will develop cancer. This process usually takes several years but sometimes can happen in less than a year. For most women, pre-cancerous cells will remain unchanged and go away without any treatment. But if these pre-cancerous cells are treated, almost all true cancers can be prevented.

> **It has been estimated that up to 80% of all sexually active women will be exposed to HPV during their lives.**

Since the most common form of cervical cancer starts with pre-cancerous changes, there are 2 ways to stop this disease from developing. The first way is to prevent the precancers, and the second is to find and treat precancers before they become cancerous.

The good news is... the U.S. Food and Drug Administration recently approved a vaccine to prevent cervical cancer. The vaccine is approved for females 9 to 26 years old. This vaccine can only be used to prevent HPV infection, before an abnormal Pap test result occurs. It cannot be used to treat an existing infection.

To be most effective, the HPV vaccine should be given before a person becomes sexually active. The American Cancer Society (ACS) also recommends that the vaccine be routinely given to females ages 11 to 12 and as early as age 9, at the discretion of doctors. The ACS recommends "catch-up" vaccinations for females ages 13 to 18. Women ages 19 to 26 should talk to their health care providers about whether to get the vaccine, based on the risk of previous HPV exposure and potential benefits from vaccination.

It is important to realize that the vaccine doesn't protect against all cancer-causing types of HPV, so routine Pap tests, as discussed in the section below, are still necessary. One other benefit of the vaccine is that it protects against the 2 viruses that cause 90% of genital warts.

Like most other cancers, cervical cancer can be treated effectively if diagnosed early. Common treatment options include surgery and chemotherapy. But the most-effective way to deal with cervical cancer is to prevent HPV from causing it.

What You Can Do

Prevent cervical cancer by having a regular Pap test to detect HPV and precancers. Treatment of precancers may stop cervical cancer before it is fully developed.

The American Cancer Society recommends the following guidelines for early detection:

All women should begin cervical cancer testing (screening) about 3 years after becoming sexually active, but no later than 21 years of age. Testing should be done every year.

Beginning at age 30, women who have had 3 normal Pap test results in a row may get tested every 2 to 3 years, or as directed by their doctor. Women who have certain risk factors such as diethylstilbestrol (DES) exposure before birth, HIV infection or a weakened immune system due to organ transplant, chemotherapy, or chronic steroid use should continue to be tested yearly.

Women 70 years of age or older who have had 3 or more normal Pap tests in a row and no abnormal Pap test results in the last 10 years may choose to stop having cervical cancer testing. Women with a history of cervical cancer, DES exposure before birth, HIV infection or a weakened immune system should continue to have testing as long as they are in good health.

Women who have had a total hysterectomy (removal of the uterus and cervix) may also choose to stop having cervical cancer testing, unless the surgery was done as a treatment for cervical cancer or precancer. Women who have had a hysterectomy without removal of the cervix (simple hysterectomy) should continue to follow the guidelines above.

Some women believe that they do not need exams by a health care professional once they have stopped having children or are menopausal. This is not correct. They should continue to follow the American Cancer Society guidelines.

Opal & diamond pendant.
A precious heirloom gift
from my grandmother.

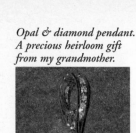

Patent mules... my "meet people"
shoes. I share but you have to
be a size 10!

White vase – reminds me of life;
beautiful, delicate and fragile

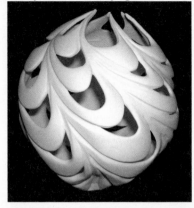

Scarf made in
Puolo, Kona
where we were
married

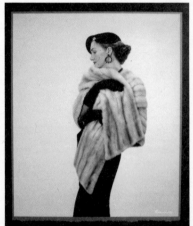

TAKE
AN
ADDITIONAL
50%
OFF
SALE ITEMS

I LOVE sales in boutiques...

My mom – a top couture model
in the 40s & 50s

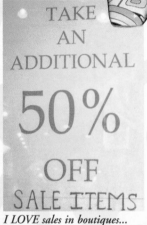

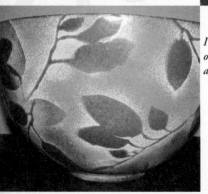

I'm a Leo, love
orange and red
and fire colors

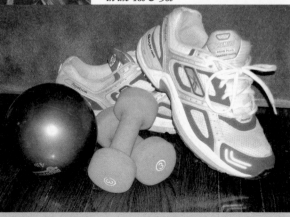

Daily
workout gear
...trusted pals

A FEW OF MY
Favorite Things

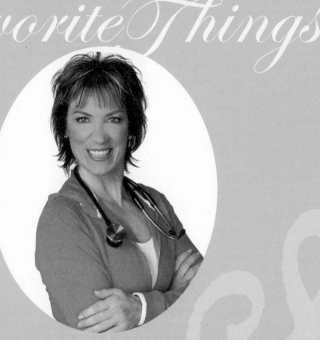

Pam Peeke, MD, MPH, FACP

Author & Speaker ~ Peeke Performance

"This sculpture is called 'Sunny Mama.' She spins around on that little rod on that one leg. I got her at a Georgetown gallery here in Washington DC. I keep her on my desk at all times. No matter what happens in my life, I simply look at her and she brings 'Sun' into my mood and my life. Sometimes I just make her spin around and around, especially when something wonderful has just happened. Such is Sunny Mama."
And we say, *"Such is Dr. Pam Peeke!!"*

Healthy Transitions

If your favorite thing is getting your period... okay, we're kidding!

Many women say that one of the best things about menopause is no more cramps, no more bloating, no more excessive moodiness... okay, you get it. Mention the word menopause in a room full of women, and just watch the eyes roll. The important thing to remember is that like puberty, pregnancy and peri-menopause, menopause itself is a natural transition we will all experience. Many women describe menopause as the beginning of a liberation from pregnancy worries and monthly periods. It signals a time of wisdom, maturity and self-assurance.

For most women, menopause occurs during a time in life when there is finally a chance to focus on YOU! Perhaps the kids are out of school and the household and its daily rhythms are slowing after 20-plus years of chaos. Take advantage of this time to do the things you always promised yourself you would do!

- **Enjoy your relationships.** Take time each week to visit and talk with your girlfriends.

- **Take up a new hobby.** Pursue that drawing or pottery class you've often dreamed of.

- **Get active!** Set aside time each day for activity that you enjoy — walk with your spouse after dinner, meet a group of friends for a morning hike, try a Yoga class or get sassy with a Latin dance night!

- **Enjoy the grandkids!** Have fun exploring your community through the eyes, ears and laughter of your grandchildren. This is a way to be in touch with the joys of childhood.

- **Hit the road!** Create adventures by visiting the places you've dreamed of and imagined... whether an hour or a day away... experience new environments, cultures and cuisines and enjoy!

- **Rediscover your sexuality!** While menopause may signal physical changes such as vaginal dryness (you may consider a vaginal lubricant) and a weakening of your pelvic floor muscles... take time to explore your new self. Learn to love and accept your mature body as a stepping stone to satisfying sexual pleasure.

- **Most women have their periods for an average of 28 years.** Women commonly experience the symptoms of menopause for 2 to 5 years, and most will live one-third of their years beyond menopause! Don't think of menopause as the end... it's just a new beginning!

Take these steps to help reduce or prevent the effects of common menopausal symptoms:

- **Cool down hot flashes.** Get regular exercise, dress in layers and try to pinpoint what triggers your hot flashes. For many women, triggers may include hot beverages, spicy foods, alcohol, hot weather and even a warm room.
- **Optimize your sleep.** Avoid caffeine and plan to exercise during the day, although not right before bedtime. Relaxation techniques, such as deep breathing, guided imagery and progressive muscle relaxation, can be very helpful.
- **Strengthen your pelvic floor.** Pelvic floor muscle exercises, called Kegel exercises, can improve some forms of urinary incontinence.
- **Eat a balanced diet.** It should include a variety of fruits, vegetables and whole grains and that limits saturated fats, oils and sugars.
- **Don't smoke.** Smoking increases your risk of heart disease, stroke, osteoporosis, cancer and a range of other health problems. It may also increase hot flashes and bring on earlier menopause. It's never too late to benefit from stopping smoking.

Just as there is help to manage PMS... there are also many things you can do to ease menopausal discomfort.

Technically, menopause is the stopping of periods for an entire year. The average age is 52; however, a woman's menopause can occur at any point between her 30s and her 60s. Peri-menopause is usually the 2 to 5 years beforehand. Menopausal symptoms can range from mild nighttime sweats to "flashes" of hot and sometimes cold, both day and night. Some women spot for a few months, others may bleed occasionally for years. These symptoms are caused by hormonal fluctuations and imbalance. And there are things you can do to help. Adjusting diet, exercise and sleep patterns does work.

While menopause itself requires no medical treatment, you may need help relieving your symptoms and preventing chronic conditions that may occur with aging.

As always, exercise regularly. Get at least 30 minutes of moderate-intensity physical activity on most days to protect against cardiovascular disease, diabetes, osteoporosis and other conditions associated with aging. Exercise can also help reduce stress.

Schedule regular checkups. Talk with your doctor about how often you should have mammograms, Pap tests, lipid level (cholesterol and triglyceride) testing, DEXA (bone density) and health screening tests. (See page 140 for health screening recommendations.)

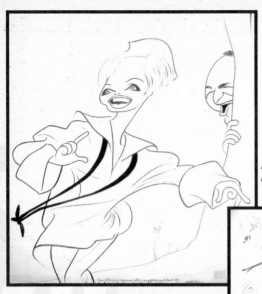

My caricature
by Hirshfeld

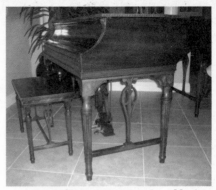

My piano

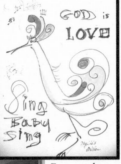

From my dear
friend, Phyllis Diller

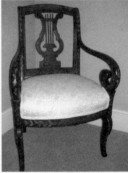

The first
antique
I ever bought

A gift for my garden
from my dear friends
Elaine and David
Marmel

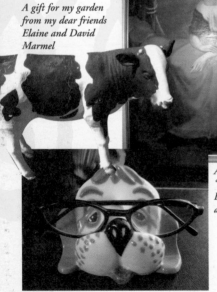

A painting of me as
"Fanny," my first
Broadway Musical
at age 19

My glasses holder

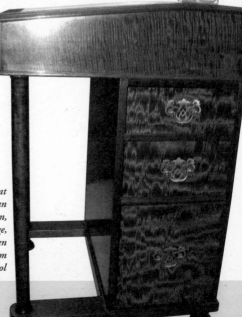

An antique desk that
once belonged to an
amazing woman,
Dr. Elsie A. George,
one of the first women
to graduate from
Columbia Medical School

A FEW OF MY
Favorite Things

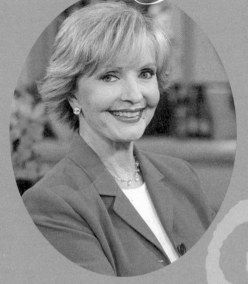

Florence Henderson

National Honorary Chair and Celebrity Spokeswoman ~ Speaking of Women's Health
Star of Stage, Screen & Television

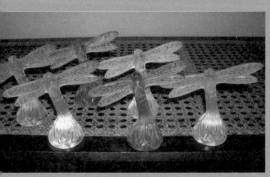

The dragonflies

"One day I was missing my late husband terribly and several dragonflies appeared in my garden. Now they are my favorites and seem to be everywhere, so I always feel his presence."

Strong Bones

If one of your favorite things is being a strong woman, this chapter is just for you.

Strong women have strong bones. Think of your bones as a framework to build upon. This chapter is chock full of news you can use about building and maintaining strong bones throughout your life.

Osteoporosis is a disease that causes bones to become thinner and more likely to break. Women's bones are strongest at about age 35 but can become weaker with age. Menopausal women can lose bone density at a faster rate and osteoporosis can result. Osteoporosis can leave all bones, especially the spine, wrist, hip and shoulder at risk for fracture. So exercise, eat calcium-rich foods and, if your doctor prescribes one, take a prescription medication.

Osteoporosis is incredibly common. A woman's risk of developing it rises with age, especially in the first 5 to 7 years after menopause. During this time, drops in estrogen may result in a 20% loss of bone mass. For women older than 50, the risk of suffering an osteoporosis-related bone fracture is about 50%. Complications from an osteoporosis-related hip fracture may be so serious as to even lead to death. Why? Immobility has been linked to blood clots, pneumonia and other concerns.

Let's Look At The Facts...

Who's at risk for osteoporosis?

- Females are more at risk than males.
- Women with blonde hair, blues eyes, a small frame and thin body (under 127 pounds).
- Those with a family history of osteoporosis.
- Women who are post-menopausal.
- Those of Caucasian or Asian race are at greater risk, but African-American and Latino women are also at risk for developing the disease.
- Those whose history includes an abnormal absence of menstrual periods or an eating disorder, such as anorexia nervosa or bulimia, which can cause menstrual periods to stop before menopause.
- Those with a diet low in dairy products or other sources of calcium and Vitamin D.
- Those with an inactive lifestyle.
- Those with a history of long-term use of certain medications (corticosteroids prescribed for many diseases, including arthritis, asthma and lupus); anti-seizure medications; gonadotropin releasing hormone for treatment of endometriosis; aluminum-containing antacids; certain cancer treatments; and excessive thyroid hormone. Talk to your pharmacist to see if your medications put you at increased risk.
- Those who smoke and overuse alcohol.

How Do I Know If I Have Weak Bones?

There are tests you can get to find out your bone strength, also called bone density.

One test is a dual-energy X-ray absorptiometry (DEXA). A DEXA takes X-rays of your bones. There are also other types of screenings to determine bone mass. Look for free screenings available in your community.

What Can You Do to Improve Your Bone Health?

Eat foods like yogurt, spinach, fortified cereals, salmon and almonds — all are calcium-rich and low in fat.

Improve muscle strength through daily weight-bearing exercise such as walking, working with hand weights, gardening or dancing.

Increase your balance by stretching your muscles daily to promote greater flexibility that leads to balance. Try Yoga or Tai Chi to help get started.

Stop smoking.

Limit alcohol intake.

Dietary Suggestions for Strong Bones:

Calcium is necessary for strong bones. This is why most women need to take a calcium supplement. Since your body can only absorb a little more than 600 mg of calcium at a time, you may need to take your supplement more than once a day. For calcium to be absorbed in the body, it needs to be combined with Vitamin D. Check the labels on your calcium supplement to ensure the ingredients are listed. To get the needed amount of calcium from your diet alone, you would need to consume:

- **Milk** – 5 glasses of milk a day

- **Yogurt, plain** – 4 cups of yogurt a day

- **Broccoli** – 8 cups of broccoli a day

Unless you are unusually fond of broccoli, most health care providers recommend a supplement.

Preventing falls and fractures is key to maintaining quality of life for women with osteoporosis. Prevent your risk of falls:
- wear sensible shoes with gripping soles
- grasp handrails on steps and inclines
- minimize the use of throw rugs in your home
- take caution when walking a pet on a leash

Sources of Calcium in Foods

Vitamin A and Beta Carotene: Sources include deep orange fruits, winter squash, carrots, broccoli, dark green leafy vegetables, liver, low-fat milk, eggs

Calcium: Low- or non-fat dairy products, broccoli, dark green leafy vegetables, sardines and salmon with bones, calcium-fortified foods

Vitamin D: Fatty fish, such as herring, salmon and sardines, egg yolks, fortified milk, fortified cereals

Vitamin K: Broccoli, Brussels sprouts, dark green leafy vegetables, liver, legumes, eggs

Manganese: Pineapple, sweet potatoes, spinach, chick peas, whole grains, brown rice, nuts, seeds

Phytoestrogens: Flaxseed, edamame (green soybeans boiled in their pods), other soy products

Zinc: Lean meats, liver, seafood, poultry, lentils, whole grains, wheat germ, buckwheat, Brazil nuts

A recent study conducted in Australia suggests that drinking tea, particularly green tea, may help maintain bone mineral density. Why? "Tea-derived flavonoids and lignans have a positive impact on osteoblast formation, which leads to stronger bones."

Source: *American Journal of Clinical Nutrition*

To learn more about osteoporosis, visit www.speakingofwomenshealth.com and type "osteoporosis" in the search box. Here you'll find more in-depth information including age-appropriate calcium and Vitamin D intake, and medications to help build and maintain strong bones and prevent osteoporosis.

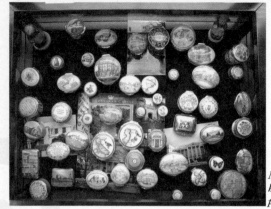

My collection of
hand-painted
porcelain boxes

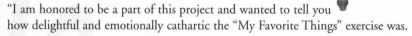

Kittinger table from the 20s,
which had belonged to
my grandmother

"I am honored to be a part of this project and wanted to tell you how delightful and emotionally cathartic the "My Favorite Things" exercise was.

When I was roaming my home doing the photography, I was surprised by how many treasures I kept around me and about the intensity of feeling associated with them. I also had my husband and daughter do their version of favorite things as well, which created a lot of laughter and some tears, too. When I spoke with my sister, she remarked that I always played the historian growing up, collecting the markers of family traditions, shared experiences and the meaningful relationships which shaped our lives.

This is a great exercise in valuing both diversity and inclusion and we will incorporate some of the ideas of "favorite things and identity" into our Women's Network activities as a way of getting to know the important women who support you in your work life.

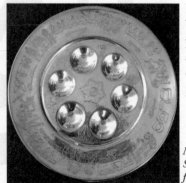

I attended a Universal Sisters (Speaking of Women's Health) Women of Color program in NYC at Columbia University last year with Dottie Peoples. It was one of the most emotionally satisfying days I have ever spent. Your organization and its commitment to women is unparalleled. We at Stryker are all very proud to be partners/sponsors with Speaking of Women's Health.

My mother's sterling silver
Seder plate, which she received
from her grandmother

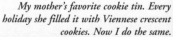

My mother's favorite cookie tin. Every
holiday she filled it with Viennese crescent
cookies. Now I do the same.

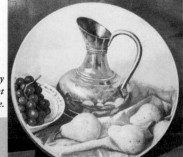

A FEW OF MY
Favorite Things

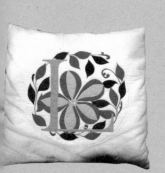

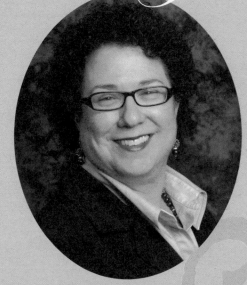

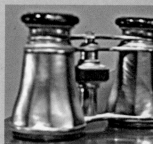

I love going to the Met, especially to see Tosca and la Boheme. These mother-of-pearl opera glasses with the lilac tint were from my dear friend Pat who is now deceased.

Lisa Peterson
Vice President, HR Practices - Stryker

Coach quilted purse. This makes me very happy, especially the purple squares!

Loet Vanderveen bronze animals, a gift from my in-laws

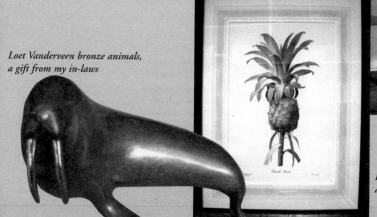

Bromelia ananas by P.J. Redouté, a gift from my husband

Keep Your Joints Jumpin'

If your favorite things include dancing, sports, even playing with your kids or grandkids, the pain of arthritis may keep you from enjoying these activities. But don't despair... this chapter will help you find solutions to enjoy your favorite things.

The term "arthritis" encompasses more than 100 diseases and conditions that affect joints, the surrounding tissues and other connective tissues. Arthritis can cause mild to severe pain in the joints, as well as tenderness and swelling.

The various forms of arthritis and related conditions can affect anyone, no matter what your race, gender or age. 60% of all people who have arthritis are female and several of the more common forms are more prevalent in women.

Osteoarthritis (OA), also known as degenerative joint disease, is the most common form of arthritis. Women usually develop OA after age 40. It causes damage to cartilage and bones, resulting in joint pain, swelling, stiffness and loss of function. Arthritis-related joint problems include pain, stiffness, inflammation and damage to joint cartilage (the tough, smooth tissue that covers the ends of the bones, enabling them to glide against one another) and surrounding structures. Such

> **The various forms of arthritis and related conditions can affect anyone, no matter what your race, gender or age.**

damage can lead to joint weakness, instability and visible deformities that, depending on the location of joint involvement, can interfere with the most basic daily tasks such as walking, climbing stairs, using a computer keyboard, cutting your food or brushing your teeth.

Rheumatoid arthritis (RA) usually strikes women between the ages of 25 to 50, but can occur in children. RA is a systemic disease that can affect the entire body. An abnormality in the body's immune system causes it to work improperly, leading to inflammation in the lining of the joints and other internal organs. Chronic inflammation can lead to deterioration, pain and limited movement. More than 2 million American adults have RA, with women outnumbering men 3 to 1.

One of the most exciting changes in recent years has been the growing understanding that the patient has an important role to play in the management of arthritis.

If you have pain, stiffness or swelling in or around a joint for more than 2 weeks, it's time to see your doctor. These symptoms can develop suddenly or slowly. Only a doctor can tell if it's osteoarthritis. Here's what you can do:

- **Exercise** helps lessen pain, increases range of movement, reduces fatigue and helps you feel better overall. Exercise regularly with non-impact activities such as water aerobics, swimming, walking, Yoga or weight-bearing strength training.

- **"C" your way to health.** Recent research has shown the importance of Vitamin C and other antioxidants in reducing the risk of osteoarthritis and its progression.

- **Learn something new about arthritis.** Building an understanding of your disease is an important step in managing it. Log on to **www.speakingofwomenshealth.com** to learn more and to stay informed.

- **Laugh, often.** It has been found to relax muscles, relieve pain and even boost your immune system.

- **Maintain a healthy weight.** You won't just look better, you'll feel better, too. Why? Every extra pound you carry translates to added stress to your knees and hips.

- **Talk to your doctor** to develop a treatment plan, including prescribed medications to provide relief, both short- and long-term. In the past two years, the FDA has approved several drugs for rheumatoid arthritis, osteoarthritis and other arthritis-related diseases.

- **Talk to your pharmacist** about over-the-counter options specially formulated for joint pain relief.

- **Wear sensible shoes that fit properly.** A well-padded, well-fitting shoe with plenty of room for your toes — and their imperfections — can make a world of difference in the way your feet feel.

- **Take a warm bath before bed.** This can relieve muscle tension, ease aching joints and help you get a good night's sleep. Consider heat therapy or soothing massage at bedtime.

- **Try low impact activities with a focus on flexibility and balance** such as Yoga or Tai Chi. Take a class or start with a DVD in your home to learn the basics.

- **Apply something cold when joints are hot and inflamed.** This can decrease pain and swelling by constricting blood vessels and preventing fluids from leaking into surrounding tissues. A fun ice pack: a bag of frozen peas or corn that can be molded to the shape of your body.

- **Stop smoking.**

Joint replacement has come a long way and now more than ever is a resource to consider when other pain-relieving measures are not effective. Talk to your doctor or orthopedic surgeon to learn more about today's joint replacement, which includes less-invasive surgical options and provides a faster return to normal activities. Even artificial joints are now designed for women, not just for men.

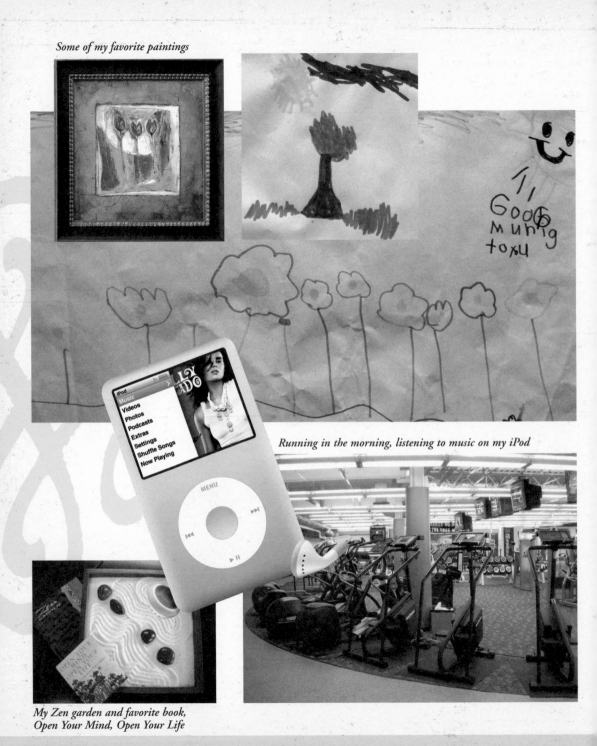

Some of my favorite paintings

Running in the morning, listening to music on my iPod

My Zen garden and favorite book,
Open Your Mind, Open Your Life

A FEW OF MY
Favorite Things

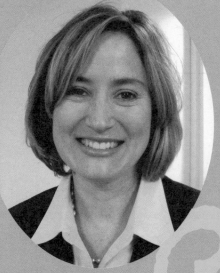

Ashley McEvoy

President, McNeil Consumer Healthcare ~ Johnson & Johnson

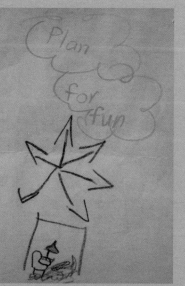

When Ashley sent back her camera with snapshots of her "favorite things," it was clear to us that this child's artwork titled, "Plan for fun" represents Ashley's philosophy of life.

Colds & Allergies

Each of us has a favorite time of year — autumn when the leaves are full of color and the sky is cornhusk blue, spring when the Earth wakes from a long winter nap, summer when the kids are playing and the pace of life slows — others enjoy winter's magic.

One thing is for sure, if you suffer the symptoms of seasonal allergies... summer, spring, winter, fall... you may need to give your pharmacist a call!

Colds or Allergies?

Because the symptoms of colds and seasonal allergies are virtually the same, it's sometimes difficult to tell which you have. Although colds and allergies may share some of the same symptoms, they are very different issues. Here's why:

Colds, also called upper respiratory infections:

- Are caused by viruses.
- Are easily spread from person to person.
- Usually last 2–14 days.
- May be prevented by frequent and thorough hand washing, and reducing exposure to others with symptoms.

Treatment may include rest, pain relievers and over-the-counter cold remedies. Check with your pharmacist.

Allergies:

- Are an immune system response caused by exposure to an allergen — something you're allergic to — such as pollen or pet dander.
- Cannot be "caught" from someone who has one.
- Have seasonal symptoms that start at the same time every year and may last for months.
- May be prevented by avoiding exposure to known allergens.

  Treatment may include over-the-counter or prescription antihistamines, nasal steroid sprays and decongestants.

The only way to truly know if you have allergies is to be tested for them in your doctor's office.

The good new is... treatment is available to help manage the symptoms of both colds and allergies. Talk to your pharmacist to help you select the appropriate over-the-counter medication to provide relief from sneezing; itchy, watery eyes; persistent cough and headache. Always take the medications only as directed.

Seasonal allergy sufferers may find relief from a variety of new medications in the form of steroid nasal sprays. These sprays won't provide immediate relief, but are designed for daily use. After about a week of use, most find a decrease in symptoms. Talk to your doctor.

Health Tips

- Wash your hands regularly to eliminate cold-causing bacteria.

- Drink 8 glasses of water daily to help rid your system of toxins.

- Eat Vitamin C-rich fruits to strengthen your immune system.

- Clean phones, keyboards and office equipment you share with others.

- Avoid close contact with people who have cold symptoms.

- Keep car windows closed to prevent pollen from collecting inside your car.

- Wash bedding weekly in hot water. Consider encasing your pillows, mattress and box springs in protective coverings made to protect from dust mites and other allergens.

- Keep pets out of the bedroom if pet dander triggers allergy symptoms.

- Reduce common indoor allergens with thorough housecleaning and consider filtering the air in your home with a HEPA filter for your furnace and vacuum cleaner. HEPA stands for High Efficiency Particulate Air-filter and can help filter pollen, mold spores, animal dander and fumes.

Symptom Checker:
Is it a cold or an allergy?

SYMPTOM	COLDS	ALLERGIES
Cough	Usually	Sometimes
General aches and pains	Sometimes	Never
Fatigue	Sometimes	Sometimes
Itchy eyes	Rarely	Usually
Sneezing	Usually	Usually
Sore throat	Usually	Sometimes
Runny nose	Usually	Usually
Stuffy nose	Usually	Usually
Fever	Rarely	Never

Source: Adapted from the National Institute of Allergy and Infectious Diseases

To help stop the spread of germs:

- Cover your mouth and nose with a tissue when you cough or sneeze.

- If you don't have a tissue, cough or sneeze into the crook of your elbow, not your hands.

- Put your used tissue in the wastebasket.

- Wash your hands with soap and water or with an instant hand sanitizer after coughing or sneezing.

Prolonged allergies that go untreated may actually weaken your immune system, putting you at higher risk for other issues including colds, flu, sinus problems and asthma. Talk to your health care provider to create an allergy action plan!

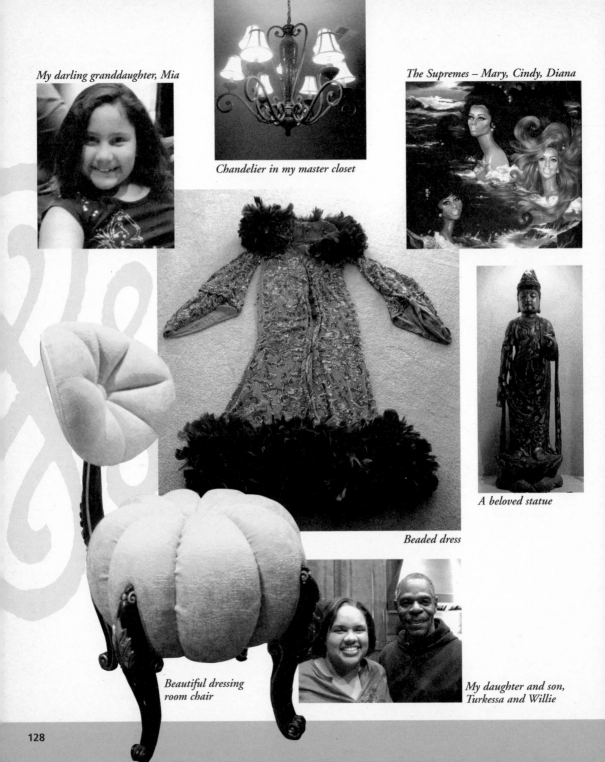

My darling granddaughter, Mia

Chandelier in my master closet

The Supremes – Mary, Cindy, Diana

A beloved statue

Beaded dress

Beautiful dressing room chair

My daughter and son, Turkessa and Willie

A FEW OF MY
Favorite Things

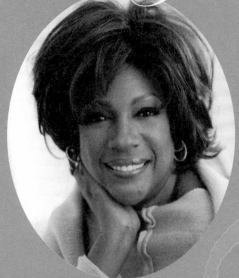

Self-portrait

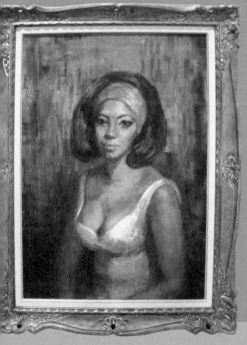

Mary Wilson

Celebrity Spokeswoman ~ Speaking of Women's Health &
Universal Sisters ~ Grammy Award-Winning Supreme

*Mary Wilson, The "Supreme" Supreme,
is an artist in every sense of the word.
Not only is Mary an iconic performing
and recording artist, as you can see
from this self-portrait, she is also a
gifted visual artist!! And... Mary is a
completely "down-to-earth girlfriend!!"*

Speaking to Men About Health™

If one of your favorite things is successfully communicating with the men in your life (while not sounding like a nag), you will love the information in this chapter.

When it comes to the men in your life, whether it's your husband, son, father, brother or friend... chances are, many women feel some responsibility for the health and well-being of these men. But, getting them to do all of the things you'd like them to do to maintain their health may be easier said than done!

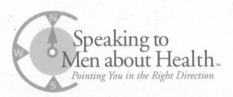

Speaking to
Men about Health™
Pointing You in the Right Direction

Tips for Speaking to Men About Health™

- Compile a routine maintenance checklist for the men in your life, including testicular and prostate self-exams, which should be done monthly.

- Teach sons to make their health and wellness a priority and to not be afraid to discuss their feelings about their health.

- Encourage your husband to put together a list of his family's health history.

- Look for ways to add more fruits and vegetables into your family's diet, maybe without them even knowing it!

- When caring for an aging male relative, make every effort to ensure that his dignity is not lost and that he is treated with respect.

Here are some tips to help women better understand how to help the men in their lives:

Understand the male approach to health.
The first step is to learn about common male feelings of fear and invincibility. Like all of us, men may fear what they don't understand and as a result of this fear, tend to ignore it.

Learn about men's health and share what you learn with him.
Seek gentle ways to share information without lecturing. For example, "I read this article about an enlarged prostate... did you know that 60% of men over the age of 60 have it?" Once you've opened a dialogue, leave an article in a place where he is likely to read it.

Compile his family's health history.
Ask his parents about their health problems because he may inherit them. Researchers are discovering many links between inheritance and the risk of disease. Compiling his family's health history will help him to identify his health priorities.

Motivate him to exercise and follow a healthy diet.
This is sometimes a challenge, but changes in diet and exercise are often most lasting when a couple adopts them together. Have fun making a date selecting a menu, going to the market, then preparing a healthy meal together.

Encourage him to share his feelings.
From an early age, men are taught to "take it like a man." The messages from society and media are strong, but a woman can go a long way toward changing this mentality by telling him it's OK to show emotions and to talk about his problems.

Find out a man's routine screening appointment schedule and post it where he can see it.
While most men know the maintenance schedule for their cars, few know how often they should visit the doctor at various ages. Also, few men know how to do self-examinations for cancers. For example, few men know that they should examine themselves each month for testicular cancer, the most common cancer in men under age 40. One survey showed that 97% of college students were unaware of this test. When a group of college students was instructed on the simple examination, 6 months later, 79% were doing it regularly.

Watch for signs and symptoms.
If a flashing red light goes off in a man's car, he will take it in for service right away. But when a warning sign goes off in his body, he may well ignore it. Women can help by knowing which symptoms are flashing red lights and by encouraging him to have them checked out right away.

Offer to accompany him.
Many men have little experience dealing with physicians. Women, who tend to be more comfortable dealing with physicians, can help a man get the most from an office visit. After a few visits, he may be more comfortable and opt to go it alone.

Help him write a list of questions.
When a doctor's appointment is essential, go to the office prepared. Studies show that, on average, a woman will ask 4 questions during a doctor's appointment; the average man asks none. Write down questions beforehand and have them ready to discuss with the doctor.

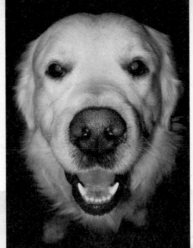

"A Dog's Smile" - Ocho, an English White Golden Retriever, is loyal, consistent and predictable in his mischief. No matter how many times, you're yelling O-C-H-O! – he melts your heart with that precocious smile.

"Breakfast Relaxation Zone" – Cabo, Mexico. I can't explain why, but there is nothing more peaceful and relaxing than Fall and Winter's sunrise and breakfast on Medano Beach. If you ever visit, see if you sip coffee and sigh, "I just don't know why watching those rocks and hearing the bark of the seals melts away stress."

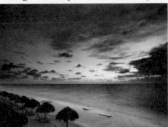

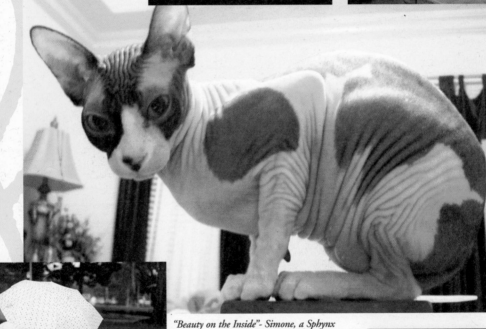

"Beauty on the Inside"- Simone, a Sphynx hairless cat, epitomizes that inner beauty is most revered and, at times, unexpected. She exhibits a "canine" personality, and is the best nighttime snuggler.

"Summer Rainy Days." Want to be a kid again?

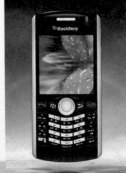

"Staying Connected" – my family embraces technology

A FEW OF MY
Favorite Things

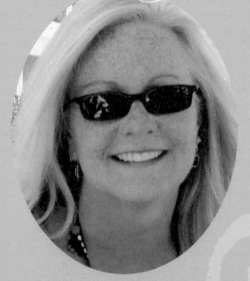

Sabrina Mills

National Sales Director, Wal-Mart Team ~ Johnson & Johnson

"Feeling of wet sand between my toes" — doesn't matter what coastline, the simple connection of warmth from the earth and heat of the sun, the melodic song of seagulls and rolling vibrations of the waves hitting the sand and resonating into my body through my toes makes me feel "one with nature" and a part of a circle of life and existence.

Personal Safety

If one of your favorite things about our motto is "Be in Charge," this chapter on personal and family safety will help make you successful.

Being informed, prepared and ready to take immediate action can put you in a powerful position in any circumstance. It can mean the difference between being confused and being confident.

While it is impossible to plan for everything, some simple precautions can help keep you and your family safe.

Be aware. Be confident. Be smart!

- Never walk with your head down. Don't stare, but always make eye contact with passersby.
- Walk with a purpose.
- Watch a person's hands as they approach you.
- Keep your keys in your hand, ready to use.
- Glance under and in your car as you approach it.
- Be aware of your surroundings. This means, parking your car in a well-lit, easy-to-find area.
- Lock your doors — house and car.
- In the summer, keep your car windows up when driving through town. Keep your purse out of sight or attached to a seat belt.
- Never stop too close to another car. You should be able to see the rear tires of the car in front of you. This will enable you to maneuver out and drive away in a threatening situation.

Safety at Home

- Equip your home with smoke and fire detectors, as well as fire extinguishers in the kitchen, garage, workshop or other areas where fire may occur. Check batteries in each detector twice a year. (NOTE: Be certain your home is free of carbon monoxide gases. At-home detectors are available.)
- Childproof your home, even if children are there just occasionally. This includes safety latches on cabinets and doors, closed doors near stairwells, childproof caps or a locked cabinet for medications, locked poisons and household detergents and child safety barriers for electrical outlets.
- Be sure all guns and firearms in your home or garage are stored in a locked cabinet. Always store bullets in a separate locked location and talk to children about gun safety at home and in other's homes.
- Teach your children to practice safe habits around animals; even if they belong to someone they know. Animals can be unpredictable. Always ask permission from the owner before approaching an animal.

Learn CPR and basic first aid, and require that regular babysitters take a basic first-aid class.

Teach your children to call 9-1-1 in the event of an emergency.

Medicine Safety

According to Wal-Mart pharmacist Karen Fruendhoff, RPH, some simple precautions will protect your family when taking medications.

- Remember that even over-the-counter medications and vitamins can cause serious problems, and even death, if a child or elderly person is overdosed.

- Only give family members medicines that have been prescribed specifically for them.

- Use the correct dose and read the label carefully.

- Follow the directions carefully and do not confuse teaspoon (tsp) with tablespoon (Tbsp). If the medicine came with a measuring device, such as a dropper, medicine cup or dosing spoon, only use it and do not substitute another device when administering it to your child. A kitchen teaspoon is not appropriate for use in measuring medication.

- If a family member is already taking a medication, make sure that any other new medicines are compatible before combining.

- Consult your pharmacist about combining prescription medications with over-the-counter drugs, including vitamins and herbal supplements.

Inventory Your Medicine Cabinet and First-Aid Kits at Least Once a Year.

- Check expiration dates. Throw out all outdated medicine. If you're not sure about a certain item, call your pharmacist and ask about the shelf life of the medicine.

- If medications are not in original containers or labeled clearly, throw them away. It's dangerous to store medicines in anything but their original containers. Some medicines come in tinted glass, for example, because exposure to light may cause deterioration.

- Every medication is a potential poison. If there are children in the house, keep all medicines and vitamins locked in a high cabinet, well out of reach.

- **If you have a poisoning emergency, call the Poison Control Hotline 1-800-222-1222 or 9-1-1.**

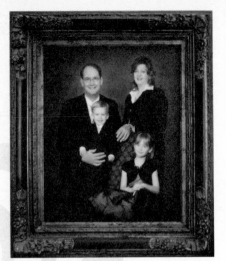

Our family portrait

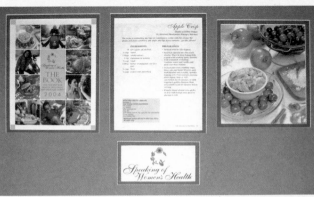

My association with Speaking of Women's Health for the past 8 years, this was my recipe in the 2004 book

This brooch, made from an antique button, was a gift from my sister, LeAnn

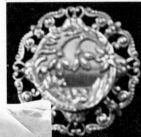

This gift from a friend and Wal-Mart associate sits in my office and reminds me of what's truly important

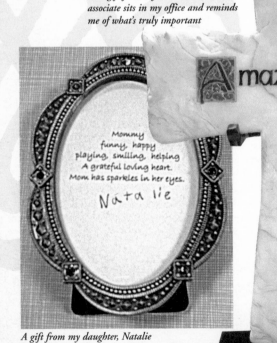

A gift from my daughter, Natalie

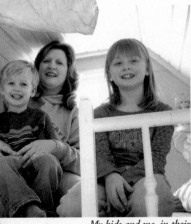

My kids and me, in their favorite place, the playhouse

A FEW OF MY
Favorite Things

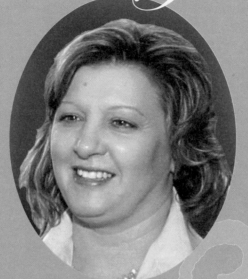

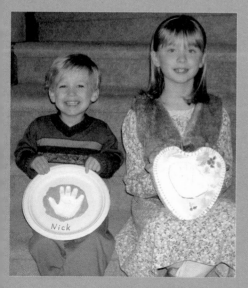

Debbie Hodges

Vice President, Logistics Asset Protection,
Compliance & Safety ~ Wal-Mart

"Out of all of these pictures, my favorite is the one of Natalie and Nicholas holding their plaster handprints that they each made for my husband, Jim and me when they were 3 years old. The handprints are priceless — but even more so were their smiles of pride when we opened the gift."

Environmental Sustainability

For many Americans, one of our most precious "favorites" is the fresh air we breathe, the clean water we drink and the beauty that Mother Nature provides.

As responsible citizens, it's imperative that we each do our part to sustain these "favorites" for future generations to enjoy. The U.S. Environmental Protection Agency (EPA) defines sustainability as "meeting the needs of the present without compromising the ability of future generations to meet their own needs." Think the efforts of one individual cannot make a difference? Think again! Do your part by incorporating these simple tips into your home and life.

Recycling Tips

- You may already recycle at home... but, what about at work? Encourage your office to begin a program. Think twice before printing e-mails. Place recycling bins around the office for recycling paper (be sure to shred confidential information first), aluminum cans and glass and printer cartridges. Ask everyone to bring in a coffee mug from home to reduce the amount of disposable cups used daily.

- Replace light bulbs with long-lasting compact fluorescent light bulbs (CFLs). It may seem like too small a change to really have any effect, but if every home in the United States just changed ONE regular light bulb to a CFL, more than a half-ton of CO_2 (carbon dioxide) would be kept out of our atmosphere. On average, a CFL uses two-thirds less energy than an incandescent light bulb. Since they last 10 times longer, CFLs are actually the most economical choice.

- Bring bags to the market, either cloth or your old paper and plastic bags. When buying only a few items, don't take a bag.

- Clean and maintain your appliances, computers, tools and cars so that they will enjoy even longer lives. And, before you replace them, check to see if they are repairable.

- Cars that receive regularly-scheduled service produce less pollution and use less energy. Check that your tires are properly inflated to ensure you're getting optimal gas mileage. Looking for a new car? Consider a hybrid that combines electricity with gas. Most average 80 miles per gallon.

- According to energy consultant Mark Jones, we already have the technology to produce cars with alternative fuel sources. What we need is the collective personal resolve to make this a reality.

- Reduce the amount of time you travel by car. Combine trips, carpool or use public transportation whenever possible.

- Replace toilets and appliances, even shower heads in your home with systems that use less water, another precious resource. Teach children to turn off the water when they brush their teeth.

- Think about composting to reduce organic waste such as plant foods (banana peels, egg shells, discarded vegetable parts, coffee grounds). These items can be stored in an air-tight container and added to your compost bin along with garden refuse, grass clippings, pine needles and leaves. The compost will eventually break down into a nutrient-rich mulch for reuse. Do not compost meat products, dairy products and high-fat foods like salad dressings and peanut butter, which can present problems. Meat scraps and the rest will decompose eventually, but will smell bad and may attract pests.

Go "Green"

A new push is sweeping the nation to go "green" to help save the planet! **The good news is...** many of these eco-friendly tips can make a positive impact on the environment and may also save you money in the long-run! Here are some tips on how to be eco-friendly in your own home:

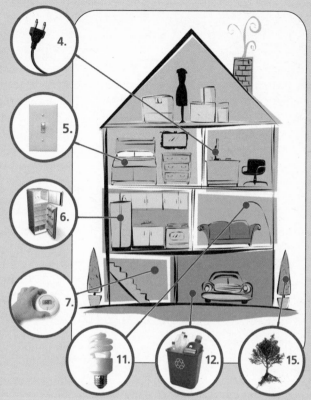

1. Set your water heater to 120°F (or lowest practical setting).

2. Use a tote bag to carry your groceries home from the grocery store.

3. Take shorter showers and install a low-flow shower head.

4. Turn off and unplug appliances when you're not using them.

5. Turn off lights in rooms when you're not home. It is a myth that turning on and off lights uses more electricity – so go ahead and turn off the lights when you leave the room!

6. Make sure your fridge and freezer temperatures aren't set too low (35-38°F for the fridge; 0°F for the freezer).

7. Set the thermostat a few degrees cooler in the winter and warmer in the summer.

8. Cancel your junk mail. Visit www.newdream.org/junkmail.

9. Wash your clothes in cold water, unless allergies are a problem.

10. Choose a highly fuel efficient, low emissions vehicle next time you buy a car.

11. Replace incandescent bulbs with compact fluorescents.

12. Recycle everything you can: school papers, paper shopping bags, soda cans, milk cartons, cereal boxes, cookie bags, foil wrap, aluminum food containers, aluminum cans, glass bottles and jars, newspapers and magazines, old cell phones and plastic water bottles.

13. Use shades and blinds to maximize heating and cooling efficiency (open shades during the day in the winter).

14. Capture rain water for your garden.

15. Plant trees to soak up carbon dioxide, help shade your home and protect it from wind.

AGE APPROPRIATE PREVENTIVE CARE TABLE

Health Activity	Ages 18-39	Ages 40-49	
Physical Exam	annually	annually	
Blood Pressure/Pulse	every other year	every year	
Eye & Ear Exam	baseline by 39	every 2-4 years	
Dental Exam	twice a year	twice a year	
Skin Exam	every 2 years	every year	
IMMUNIZATIONS			
Tetanus/Diphtheria	every 10 years	every 10 years	
Influenza (Flu)	per risk	per risk	
Measles/Mumps/Rubella	up to date	usually not needed	
Pneumonia Vaccine	usually not needed	usually not needed	
HPV	The American Cancer Society recommends the HPV vaccination for females ages 11-12 years and catch-up vaccines for females ages 13-18.		
Cholesterol/Triglycerides	at age 20	every 5 years	
Blood Sugar Evaluation (Diabetes)	usually not needed	every 3 years at 45	
Bone Density for Osteoporosis	usually not needed	usually not needed	
BREAST CANCER SCREENING			
Breast Self-Exam	teach BSE by age 20	monthly	
Mammography	usually not needed	annually	
Breast Exam by Physician	every 1-3 years	annually	
CERVICAL CANCER SCREENING			
Pap Test	The American Cancer Society recommends all women should begin cervical cancer testing (screening) about 3 years after becoming sexually active, but no later than 21 years of age. Testing should be done every year.		
Pelvic Exam by Physician	annually	annually	
COLON CANCER SCREENING			
Fecal Occult Blood Test (FOBT) or Fecal Immunochemical Test (FIT)		usually not needed	
Flexible Sigmoidoscopy		usually not needed	
FOBT or FIT, plus Flexible Sigmoidoscopy		usually not needed	
Double Contrast Barium Enema		usually not needed	
Colonoscopy		usually not needed	

Screening tests are used to identify a disease previously unrecognized, or the risk factors associated with a particular disease. A number of health care organizations publish guidelines for the use of screening tests in certain age groups. These guidelines may vary or change from time to time because of new research or differences in interpretation by different health care organizations.

Ages 50-64	Age 65+	Comments
annually	annually	as needed with health demands
every year	every year	more often with family history
every 2-4 years; 60+ yearly	yearly	more frequent visits with problems
twice a year	twice a year	as needed with changes in dental health
every year	every year	as needed with changes in skin
every 10 years	every 10 years	
yearly	yearly	pregnancy, lung disease and heart disease require immunization prior to age 50
usually not needed	usually not needed	immunity desired prior to pregnancy
usually not needed	at age 65	booster may be required in 5 years

For women ages 19-26 the vaccine should be based on an informed discussion between the woman and her health care provider. See Chapter 17 for more information.

Ages 50-64	Age 65+	Comments
every 5 years	every 5 years	more frequent if abnormality detected
every 3 years	every 3 years	*more frequent and earlier depending on risk level and family history
baseline if at risk	age 65	*may screen earlier with risk factors
monthly	monthly	always call physician with concerns
annually	annually	*risk level may require higher frequency
annually	annually	*risk level may require higher frequency

Some doctors feel that after 3 or more consecutive normal results, cervical cancer screenings may be performed every 2-3 years on certain low-risk women.

Ages 50-64	Age 65+	Comments
annually	annually	
annually	annually	
every 3-5 years	every 3-5 years	*colon screening may be performed earlier and more frequently with certain risk factors or a family history of having polyps
every 5 years	every 5 years	
every 5 years	every 5 years	
every 5 years	every 5 years	

* Your health care team can assist you in adopting screening tests that apply to your particular family history. (G. Byron Kallam, MD offers this chart as a place to begin a dialogue with your health care team.)

Index

Index

OUR HOSPITAL PARTNERS*

Speaking of Women's Health is proud to partner with these hospitals to provide the latest, most up-to-date educational resources and information. As part of our mission to "educate women to make informed decisions about health, well-being and personal safety for themselves and their families," we have partnered with these health care institutions because we feel they have shared goals and a common vision with us.

St. Anthony Medical Center, Crown Point, IN

Sarasota Memorial Health Care System, Sarasota, FL

The Women's Pavilion at St. Mark's Hospital, Salt Lake City, UT

Baptist Health, Jacksonville, FL

Tampa General Hospital, Tampa Bay, FL

St. Vincent Women's Hospital, Indianapolis, IN

Washington Regional Medical Center, Northwest AR

Shawnee Mission Medical Center, Kansas City, KS

WellStar Health System, Atlanta, GA

WakeMed Health & Hospitals, Raleigh, NC

Strong Health, Rochester, NY

Miami Valley Hospital, Dayton, OH

Cleveland Clinic Florida, Miami, FL

Mercy Hospital, Miami, FL

Virginia Commonwealth University Institute for Women's Health, Richmond, VA

University of Missouri Health Care, Columbia, MO

TriHealth Women's Health: Bethesda North and Good Samaritan hospitals, Cincinnati, OH

Boone Hospital, Columbia, MO

The Cleveland Clinic Foundation, Cleveland, OH

Sara Lee Center for Women's Health at Forsyth Medical Center, Winston-Salem, NC

King's Daughters' Hospital, Madison, IN

Margaret Mary Community Hospital, Batesville, IN

Covenant Health Systems, Waterloo, IA

Northwest Texas Healthcare System, Amarillo, TX

Orlando Regional Healthcare, Orlando, FL

Sharp Health Care System, San Diego, CA

Mercy Health Partners, Cincinnati, OH

Jackson Hospital, Montgomery, AL

Mills-Peninsula Health Services, San Mateo, CA

Capital Health Lois Hole Hospital for Women, Edmonton, Canada

Loma Linda University, Loma Linda, CA

*as of this printing